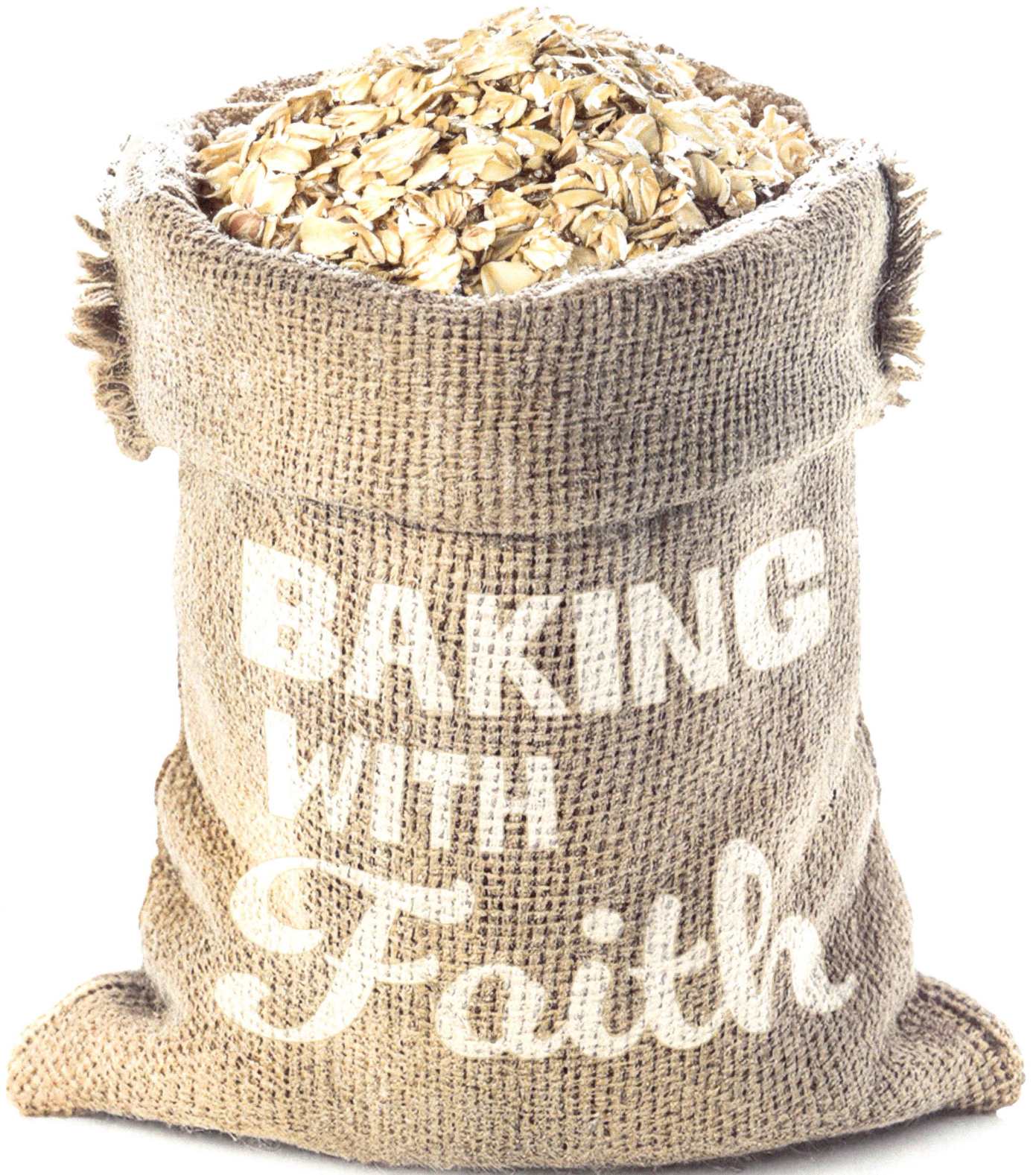

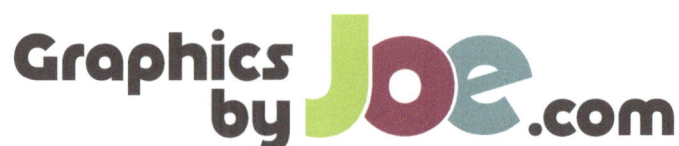

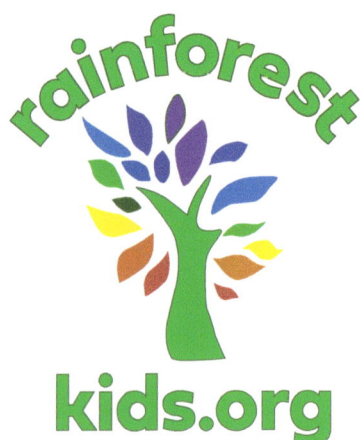

First edition: November 2024
ISBN: 979-8-9916442-2-8

WELCOME TO BAKING WITH *Faith*

Joe and I are delighted to share the most popular recipes from my bakery on Costa Rica's Pacific coast. Since I believe that baking, like life, is best when simple, I've streamlined these recipes to eliminate unnecessary fuss. Most ingredients are easily found in supermarkets anywhere, so no need to hunt in specialty stores. Plus, the recipes require only basic kitchen tools, so you won't need to buy fancy equipment. With your health and the health of the planet in mind, most recipes are vegan or can be made vegan—and they taste so good, no one will know unless you tell them!

The recipes range from super simple to a bit more complex, so beginner bakers and kids will find many easy to make. Little ones especially enjoy making the Free Cookies, with the fun of squishing bananas by hand! As you gain confidence, you can try more adventurous creations like Sourdough Bread Demystified and Sprouted Lentil Curry Veggie Burgers.

We really hope you enjoy *Baking with Faith*. Thank you for buying this book and supporting the Rainforest Kids mission for environmental education (**rainforestkids.org**). We'd love to hear your thoughts and suggestions to improve future editions!

Faith Inman

NOTES

INGREDIENTS

Flour When I say flour, I mean regular white flour made from the starchy part of wheat grains, except for when I make it clear to use whole wheat flour.

Solid fat Options here include: shortening, margarine, butter, lard, or palm oil. Use what makes sense to you.

Sugar You can use raw or turbinado sugar for everything. If the sugar is coarsely ground, it will add delightful little crystals to your cookies. But if you only have white or brown sugar, that works just fine too.

Vegetable oil Don't use olive oil for the sweets. Otherwise, any kind of vegetable oil you have on hand is fine.

Vinegar Plain white vinegar works perfectly. Red and white wine vinegar are also good. If you use apple cider vinegar, add a smidge extra to compensate for the lower acidity. Balsamic vinegar is too neutral and won't work.

PREPARATION

Bake time Baking times are approximate because ovens vary.

Mixing The beauty of these recipes is that they don't require any fancy gear. You can mix most of these recipes with a big spoon or your bare hands. The exception is the frosting. You'll need an electric mixer for that.

Pan prep To prepare baking sheets for cookies, cover them with waxed paper or silicone baking parchment. Alternatively, you can coat the baking surface with a thin layer of oil or solid fat. For cake, bread, or muffin pans, you can line them with waxed paper or cupcake liners. Another option is to grease the pans with a thin layer of oil or solid fat, then sprinkle in some flour, tap it around to coat the surface evenly, and discard any excess flour. To make your life easier, use silicone baking pans because they don't need greasing.

Yield The yield depends on the size of each cookie, muffin, and so forth.

MEASUREMENTS

tsp = teaspoon (5 ml)

Tbsp = tablespoon (15 ml)

cup = US cup (240 ml)

CONTENTS

PASTRIES

TOPPING & FROSTINGS

CAKE AND PIE

COOKIES

BREADS AND PIZZA DOUGH

BURGERS

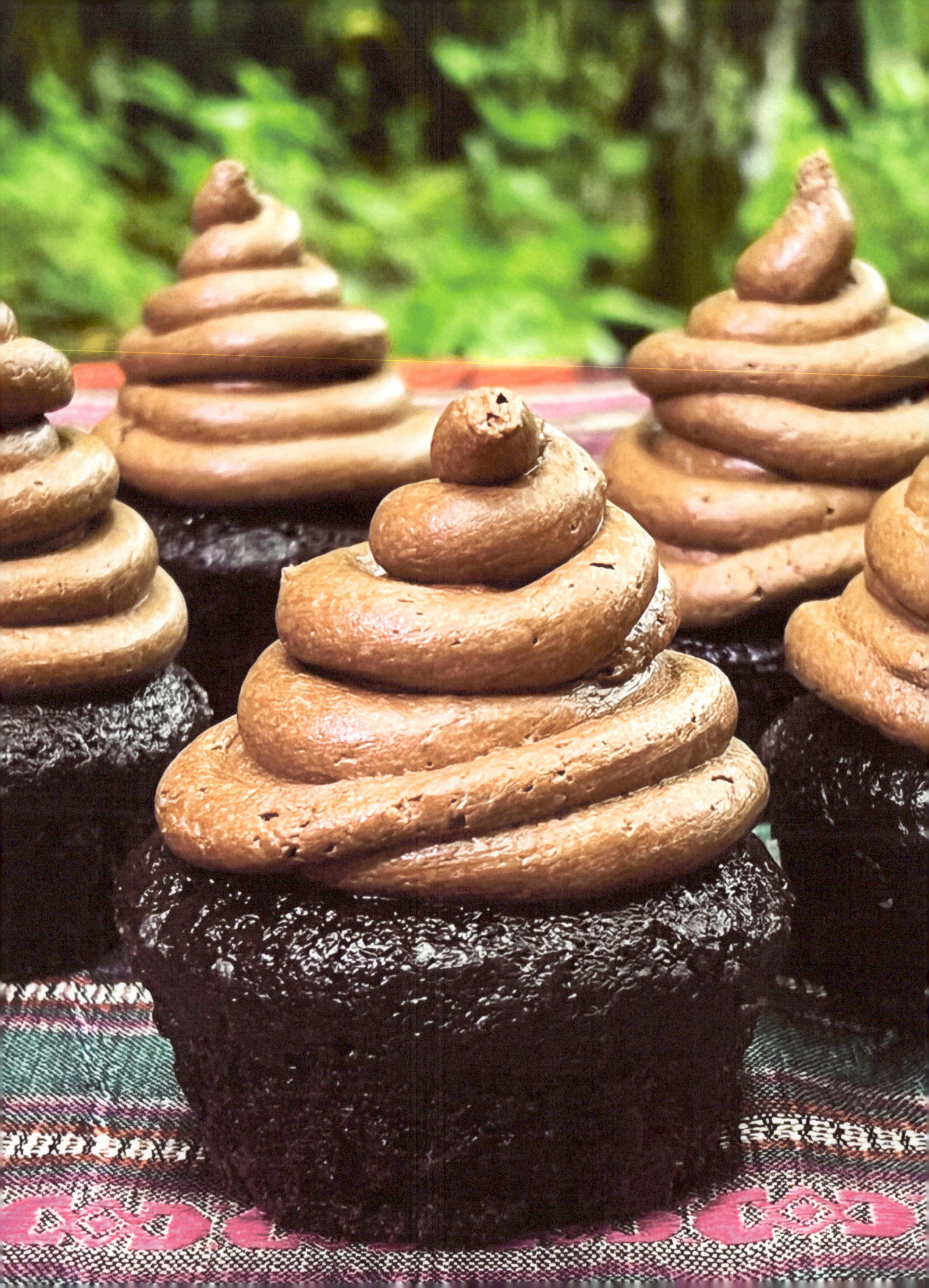

MOCHA CHOCOLATE VOLCANO CUPCAKES

Did you ever make a baking soda and vinegar volcano as a kid in science class? That's the same chemistry magic that makes these cupcakes rise.

INGREDIENTS

◇◇◇◇◇◇◇◇◇◇◇◇◇

Dry
- 1 ½ cups flour
- 1 cup sugar
- 1/2 cup cocoa powder
- 1 tsp baking soda
- 1/2 tsp salt

Wet
- 1 cup hot, strong, black coffee
- 1/2 cup vegetable oil
- 1 Tbsp vinegar
- 1 tsp vanilla

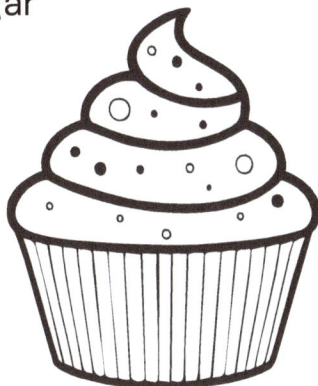

INSTRUCTIONS

◇◇◇◇◇◇◇◇◇◇◇◇◇

1. Mix the dry ingredients until evenly combined.
2. Stir the wet ingredients together, though the oil and water will stubbornly refuse to mix.
3. Combine the wet and dry ingredients until smooth. Use a spoon, whisk, or electric mixer.
4. Scoop the batter into cupcake pans prepared with liners or greased and floured. Fill each cup about 2/3 full.
5. Bake at 350°F until a toothpick inserted in the center comes out clean, about 20 minutes.
6. Allow to cool completely before frosting with **Angel Poo** or **Mocha Angel Poo Frosting**.

Notes:
Since these have coffee in them, I consider them breakfast cupcakes. Yes, that's right, I eat volcanoes for breakfast.

vegan

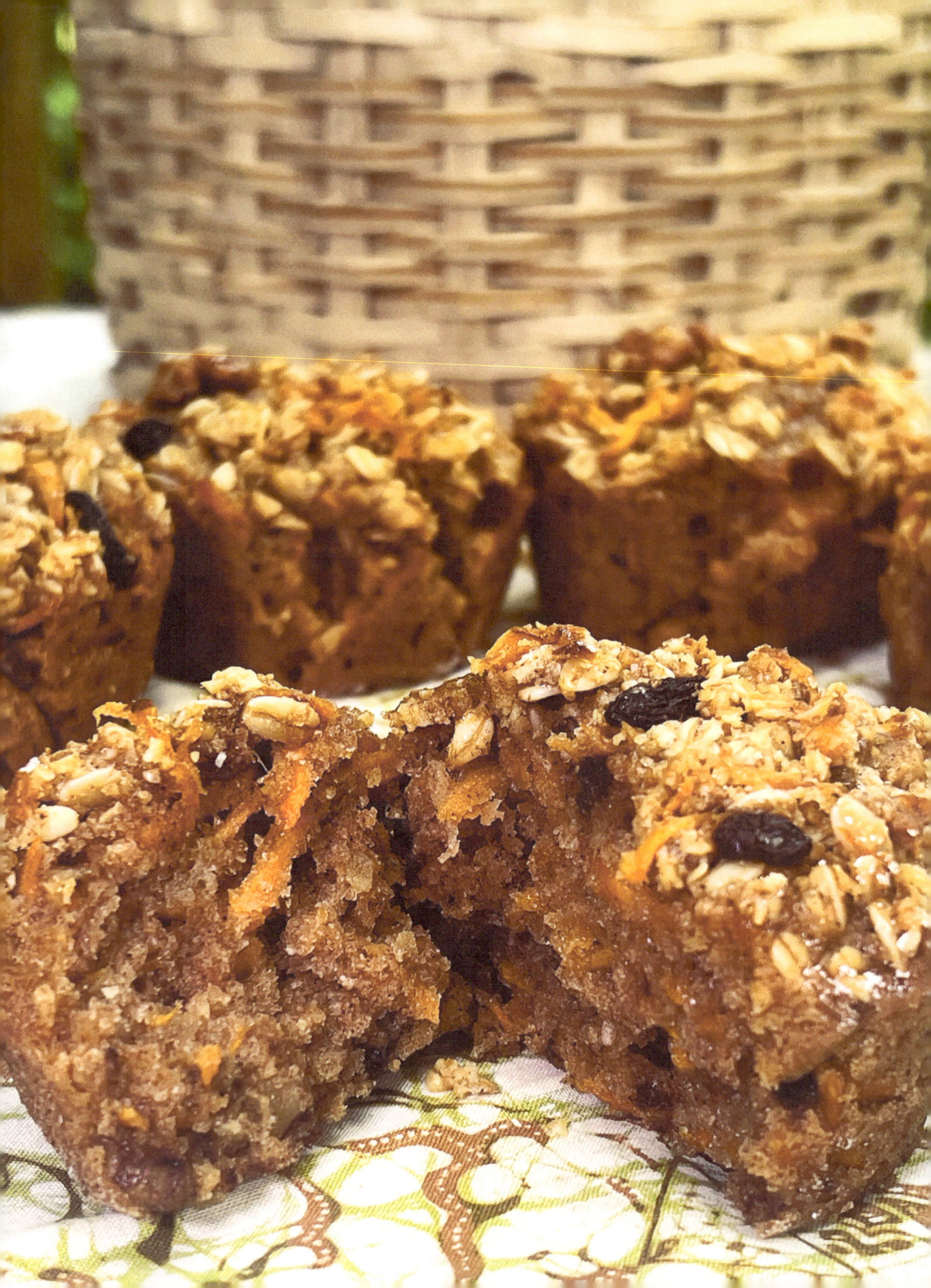

SPICY CARROT GINGER MUFFINS

Definitely not your grandma's carrot muffin. These are intensely flavored, textured, and moist muffins. Your friends will gobble these up fast.

INGREDIENTS

◇◇◇◇◇◇◇◇◇◇◇◇◇

Dry
- 1 ¾ cups flour
- 1 cup sugar
- 1 tsp baking soda
- 1/2 tsp salt
- 1 Tbsp cinnamon
- 1 Tbsp ginger

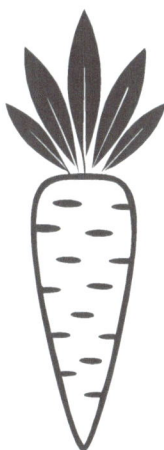

Wet
- 1 cup hot water
- 1/3 cup oil
- 1 tsp vanilla
- 1 Tbsp vinegar
- 1 cup shredded carrot
- 1 Tbsp shredded fresh ginger (if available)

INSTRUCTIONS

◇◇◇◇◇◇◇◇◇◇◇◇◇

1. Mix the dry ingredients until evenly combined.
2. Stir the wet ingredients together, though the oil and water will still refuse to mix.
3. Combine the wet and dry ingredients together, but gently to not spoil the magic.
4. Scoop the batter into muffin pans prepared with liners or greased and floured. Fill each cup about 2/3 full.
5. Bake at 350°F until a toothpick inserted in the center comes out clean, about 25 minutes.

Notes:
- Top with **Crunchy Crumble Topping** before baking for extra yum.
- Add raisins (extra nice if you soak them in the hot water to plump up), walnuts, shredded coconut (reduce the sugar if you use the sweetened kind), and/or pineapple pieces.

vegan

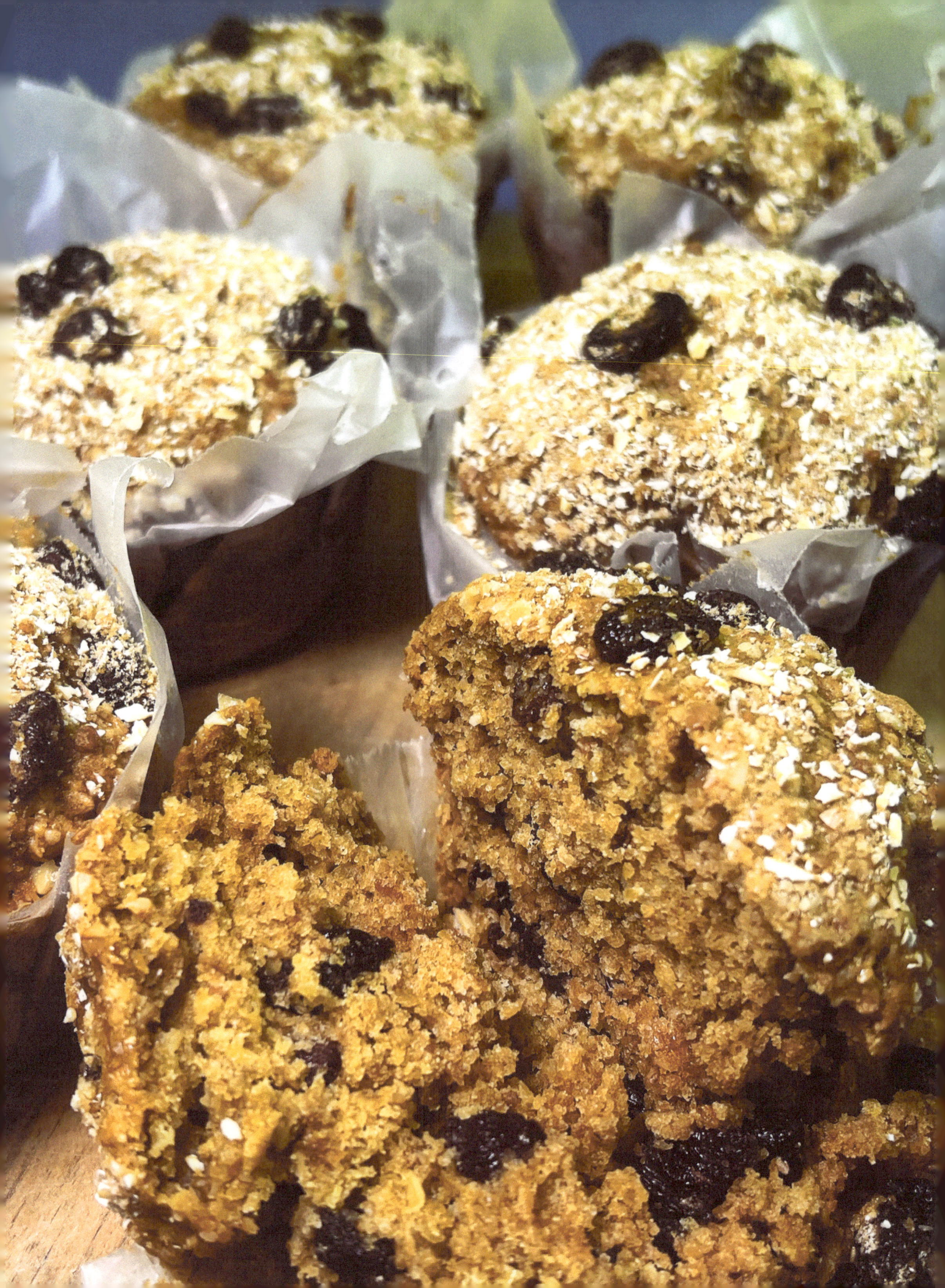

RAISIN THE BAR BRAN MUFFINS

So soft and light, with a flavor reminiscent of Raisin Bran cereal. You'll want to eat these for breakfast every morning.

INGREDIENTS

◇◇◇◇◇◇◇◇◇◇◇◇◇◇

Dry
- 1 ½ cups flour
- 1 tsp baking soda
- 2/3 cup bran
- 2/3 cup raisins

Wet
- 2/3 cup sugar
- 1/3 cup oil or solid fat
- 1/4 tsp salt
- 1 tsp vanilla
- 1 Tbsp vinegar
- 1 cup hot water

INSTRUCTIONS

◇◇◇◇◇◇◇◇◇◇◇◇◇◇

1. Mix the dry ingredients until evenly combined.
2. Blend the wet ingredients together.
3. Combine the wet and dry ingredients.
4. Scoop the batter into muffin cups prepared with liners or greased and floured. Fill each cup about 2/3 full.
5. Bake at 350°F until a toothpick inserted in the center comes out clean, about 25 minutes.

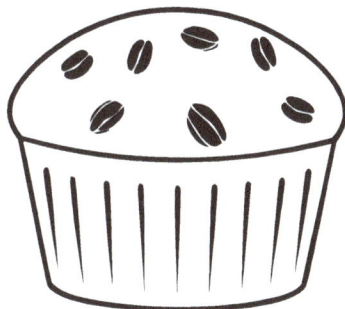

vegan

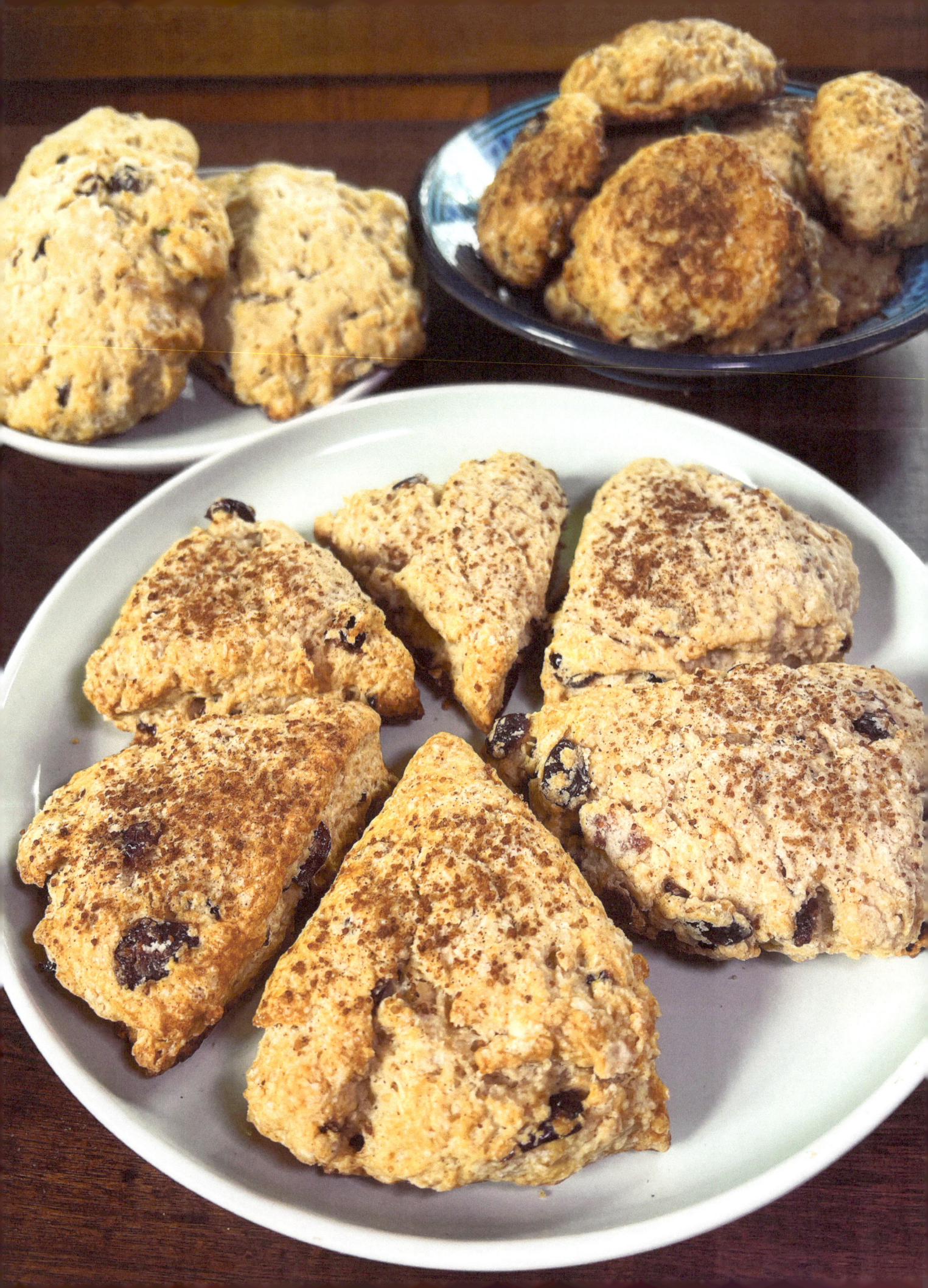

LAZY DAY CRANBERRY SCONES

My grandmother says, "Scones are just biscuits with an attitude." The secret to scones is to be lazy. Don't mix them up too much. Instead, let the dough stay loose so the scones come out crumbly. If it looks like everything is falling apart, that's when you know you've got it right.

INGREDIENTS

◇◇◇◇◇◇◇◇◇◇◇◇

Dry
- 2 cups flour
- 1/3 cup sugar
- 1 Tbsp baking powder
- 1 Tbsp ground flax seeds
- 1/2 tsp salt
- 1 tsp cinnamon
- 1 pinch nutmeg
- 3/4 cup dried cranberries

Wet
- 1/2 cup solid fat (shortening, margarine, or butter)
- 1/3 cup soy or almond milk

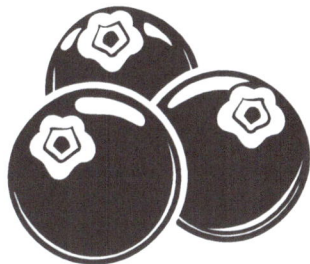

INSTRUCTIONS

◇◇◇◇◇◇◇◇◇◇◇◇

1. Mix dry ingredients.
2. Cut in fat with fingers until more or less absorbed in flour.
3. Add the milk to the dry ingredients and toss a few times until the whole mess starts to come together.
4. Dump directly onto a baking sheet covered with waxed paper or a silicone baking sheet and pat into a roughly circular form about 2 inches thick.
5. Cut into 8 wedges and pull apart to separate.
6. Sprinkle scones with cinnamon and sugar.
7. Pop into the oven and bake at 350°F until golden brown, about 20 minutes.

Notes:

Gobble these up fresh out of the oven or let them cool, slice in half, toast, and top with butter and jam. Serve with tea, obviously.

Vegan

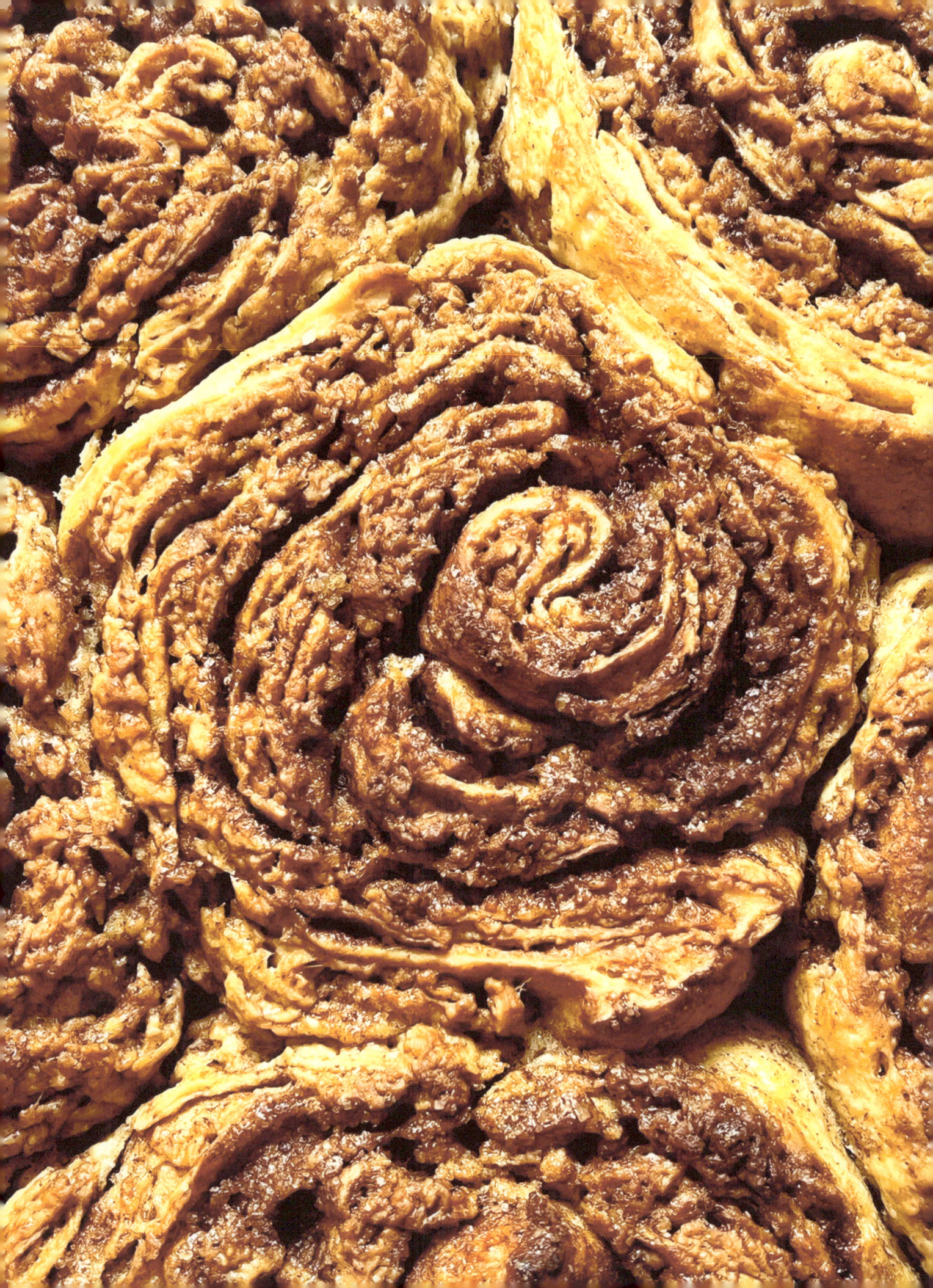

GALACTIC SPIRAL CINNAMON ROLLS

These are the best cinnamon rolls on this side of the galaxy. The other side of the galaxy has pretty good ones too, but it's a drive.

INGREDIENTS

◇◇◇◇◇◇◇◇◇◇◇◇◇

- 1 batch **Quick & Easy Pizza Dough**
- 1/2 cup solid fat (shortening, margarine, or butter)
- 1 cup sugar
- 2 Tbsp cinnamon

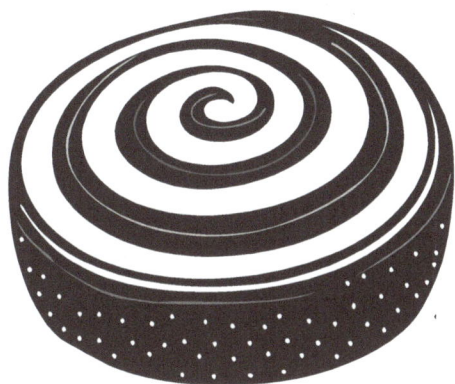

INSTRUCTIONS

◇◇◇◇◇◇◇◇◇◇◇◇◇

1. Mix the cinnamon and sugar together.
2. Pat dough into a rectangle about 1 inch thick.
3. Smear on about 1/4 of the fat to cover the dough.
4. Sprinkle on about 1/4 of the cinnamon-sugar.
5. Roll dough lengthwise into a log.
6. Repeat steps 2-5 until the fat and cinnamon & sugar are used up.
7. Cut dough log into 6-8 slices.
8. Place each slice onto a greased baking sheet and allow to rise for 20 minutes.
9. Bake at 350°F until lightly browned on top, about 25 minutes.

Notes:
Top the piping hot cinnamon rolls with **Angel Poo Frosting** to make yourself a Cinnabon-style treat at home.

vegan

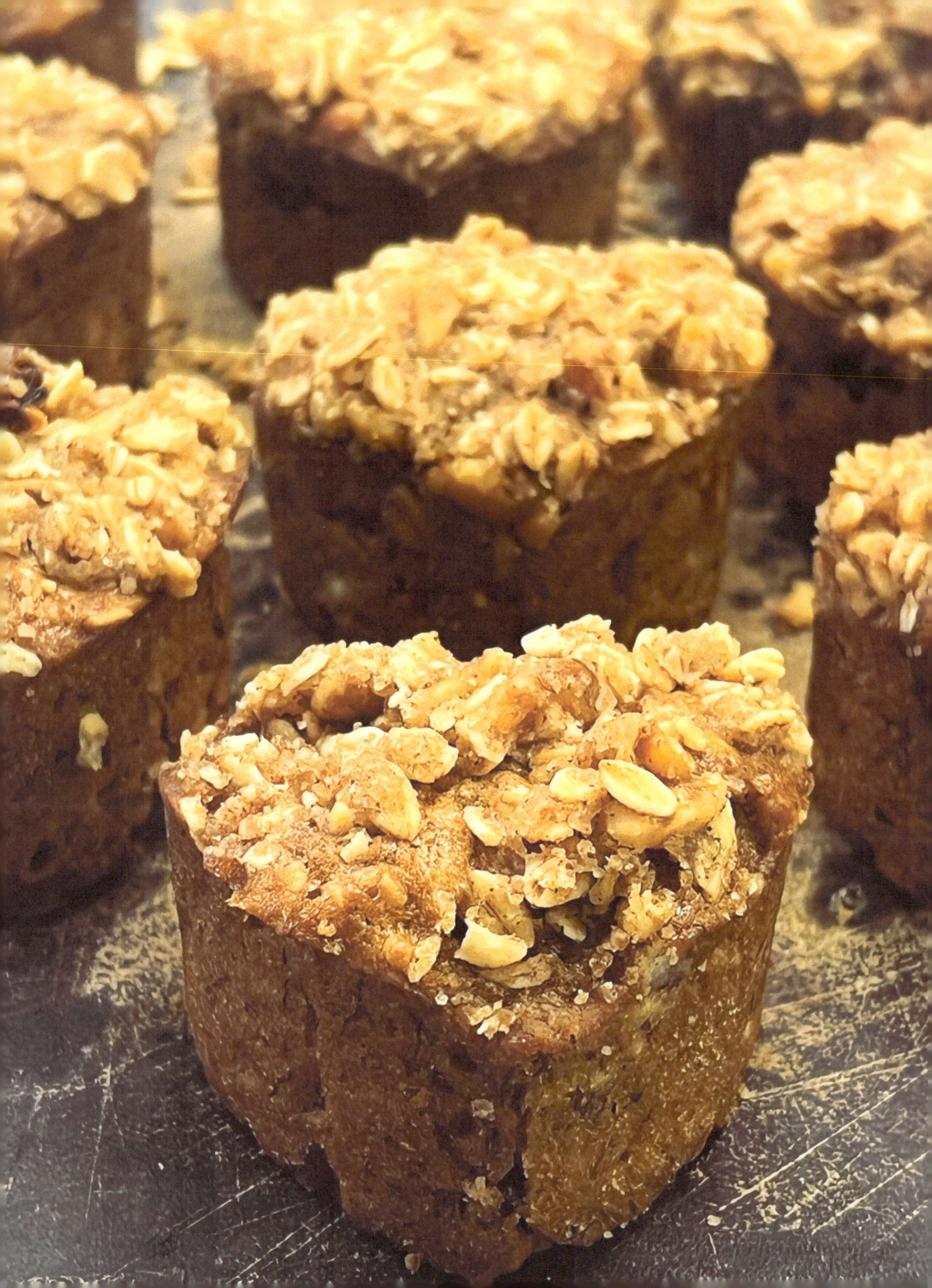

BANANA LOVE MUFFINS

My surfer buddies call these muffins "epic". They will also help you use up a few of those overripe bananas.

INGREDIENTS

◇◇◇◇◇◇◇◇◇◇◇◇

Dry
- 3 cups flour
- 1 cup old-fashioned oats
- 1 Tbsp baking soda
- 1 Tbsp cinnamon

Wet
- 1 cup sugar
- 1/2 tsp salt
- 1 cup solid fat or oil
- 1 cup water
- 3 Tbsp vinegar
- 1 Tbsp vanilla
- 3 ripe bananas

INSTRUCTIONS

◇◇◇◇◇◇◇◇◇◇◇◇

1. Mix the dry ingredients until evenly combined.
2. Blend the wet ingredients together. An electric mixer makes this easy.
3. Combine the wet and dry ingredients.
4. Scoop the batter into muffin pans prepared with liners or greased and floured. Fill each cup about 2/3 full.
5. Bake at 350°F until a toothpick inserted in the center comes out clean, about 25 minutes.

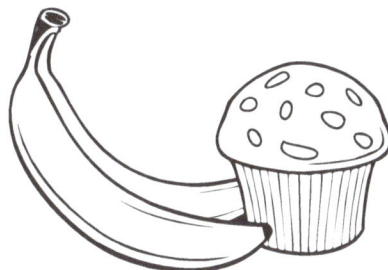

Notes:

Pile on the **Crunchy Crumble Topping** before baking. Add nuts or raisins to the batter for even more texture and flavor.

vegan

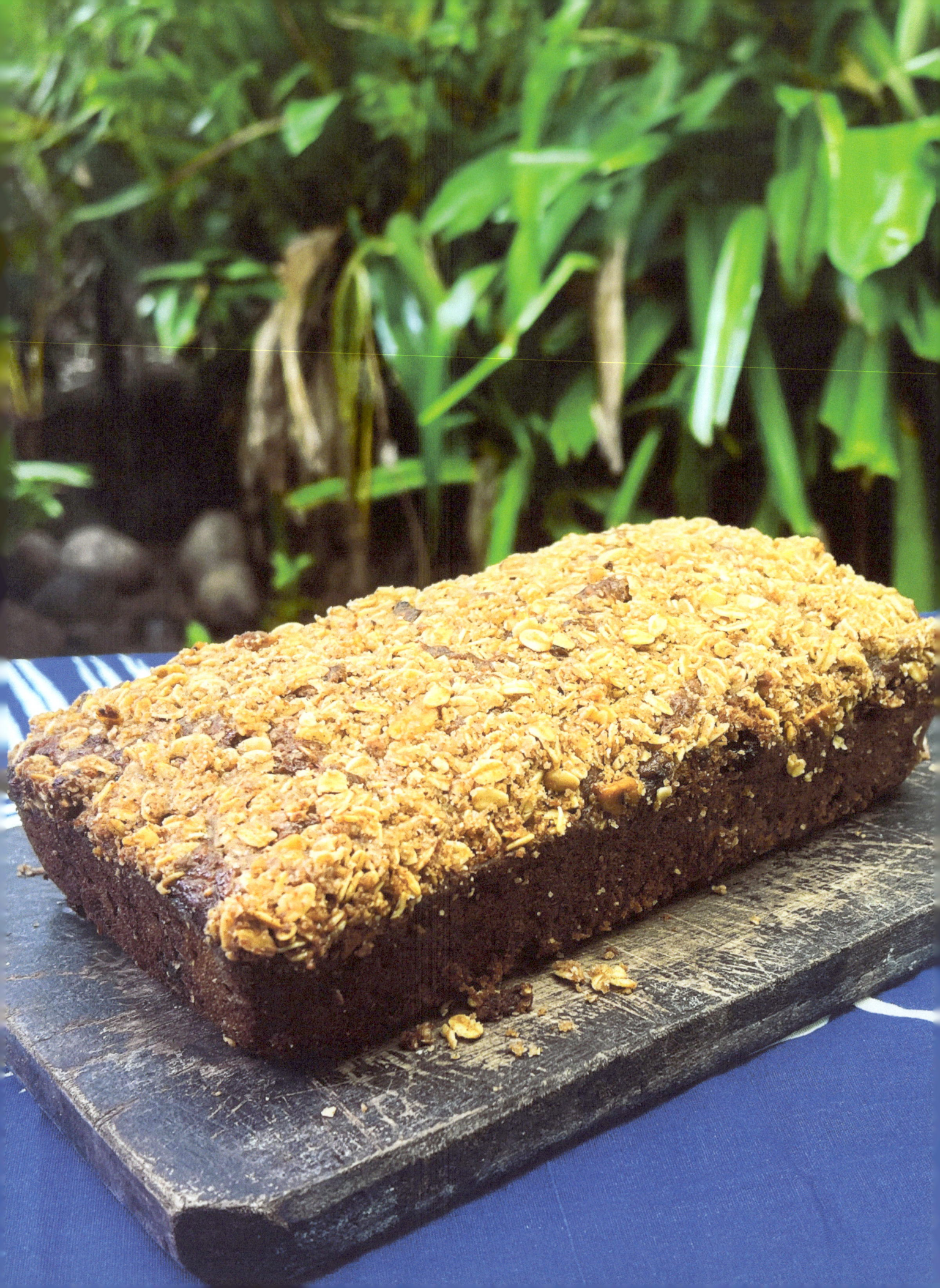

CRUNCHY CRUMBLE TOPPING

Top muffins with Crunchy Crumble Topping before baking to up your muffin game to the next level. I like to really pile on as much topping as possible to get the most crunch.

INGREDIENTS

◇◇◇◇◇◇◇◇◇◇◇◇◇◇

- 1/4 cup oil or solid fat
- 1/2 cup sugar
- 1 Tbsp cinnamon
- 1/4 tsp salt
- 1 tsp vanilla
- 1 cup old-fashioned oats
- 1/4 cup flour
- 1/2 cup chopped nuts

INSTRUCTIONS

◇◇◇◇◇◇◇◇◇◇◇◇◇◇

1. Blend all the ingredients together. An electric mixer makes this easy.
2. Put a generous amount on top of muffins or bread before baking. Press down into batter to help it stick.

Notes:
You can store the extra topping in the fridge or freezer for a while, so you have it handy for the next time you want to bake.

vegan

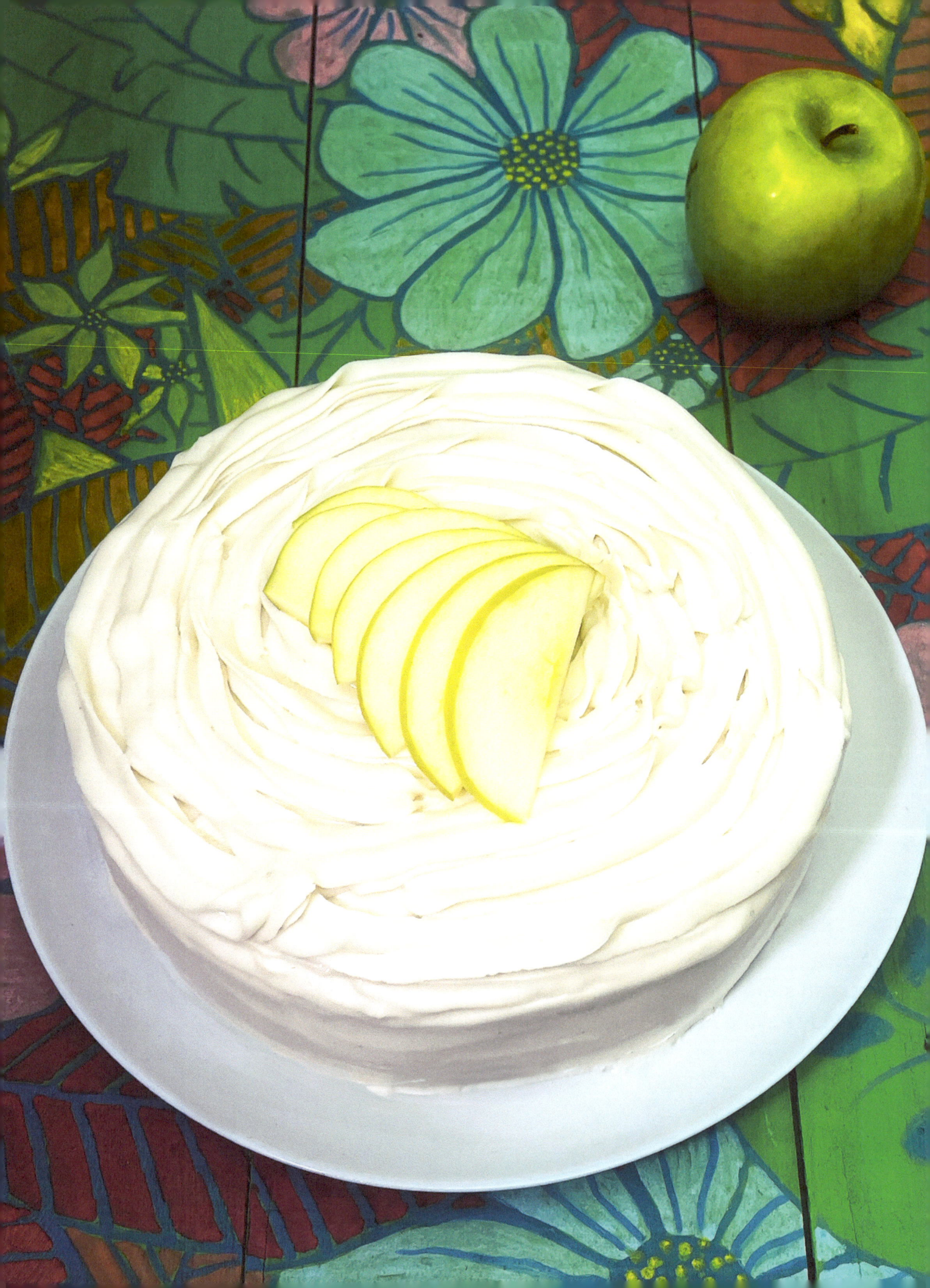

FROSTING

ANGEL POO FROSTING

INGREDIENTS

- 3 cups powdered sugar
- 1/2 cup solid fat
- 1/3 cup milk, juice, or water
- 1 tsp vanilla

INSTRUCTIONS

1. Put all the ingredients in a steep sided bowl and mix with an electric mixer until fluffy.
2. Color if desired.
3. Apply to cakes and cupcakes with a spatula or pastry bag.

MOCHA ANGEL POO FROSTING

INGREDIENTS

- 3 cups powdered sugar
- 1/2 cup cocoa powder
- 1/2 cup solid fat
- 1/3 cup cool coffee
- 1 tsp vanilla

INSTRUCTIONS

1. Put all the ingredients in a steep sided bowl and mix with an electric mixer until fluffy.
2. Apply to cakes and cupcakes with a spatula or pastry bag.

SWEET TART LEMON ICING

INGREDIENTS

- 1 cup powdered sugar
- 3-4 Tbsp lemon juice

INSTRUCTIONS

1. Mix the powdered sugar with enough lemon juice to get a good consistency.
2. Color, if desired, and pipe or paint onto cooled cookies.

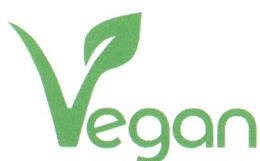

Vegan

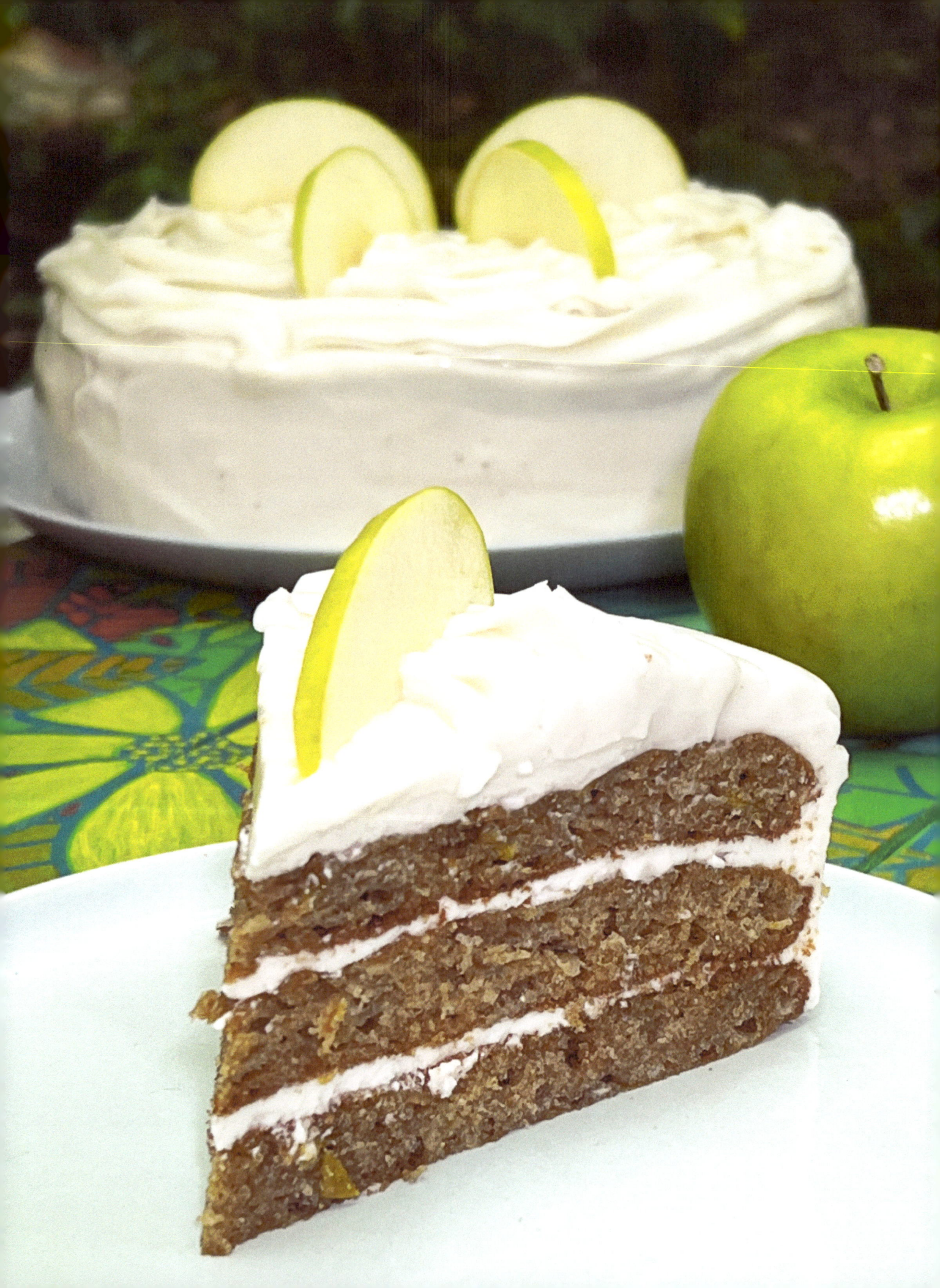

A IS FOR APPLE CAKE

Kids love this recipe – both making it and eating it! It's a fun way to learn about measurements, fractions, and baking.

INGREDIENTS

◇◇◇◇◇◇◇◇◇◇◇◇

Dry
- 1 ½ cups flour
- 1 ½ tsp baking soda
- 1 tsp baking powder
- 1 Tbsp pumpkin spice powder
  – Or 1 tsp cinnamon, 1 tsp ginger, 1/2 tsp clove, 1/2 tsp nutmeg, and 1/2 tsp allspice powders

Wet
- 1 ½ cups grated green apple
- 1 cup sugar
- 2/3 cup vegetable oil
- 1/2 tsp salt
- 3 eggs

INSTRUCTIONS

◇◇◇◇◇◇◇◇◇◇◇◇

1. Mix the dry ingredients until evenly combined.
2. Stir the wet ingredients together.
3. Combine the wet and dry ingredients.
4. Pour into greased and floured baking pans.
5. Bake at 350°F until a toothpick inserted into the center comes out clean, about 30 minutes.
6. Once the cake is completely cool, frost with **Angel Poo Frosting**.

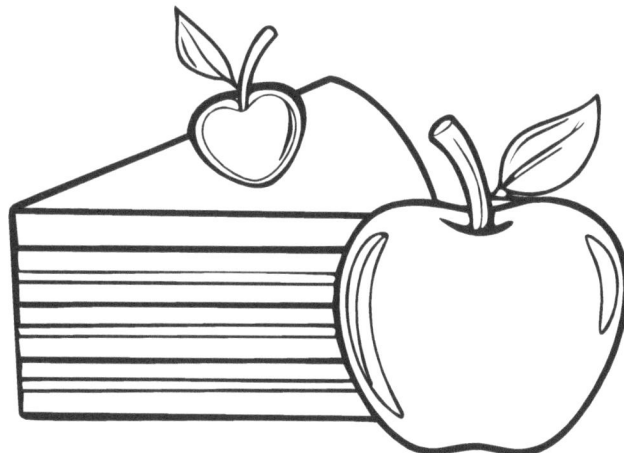

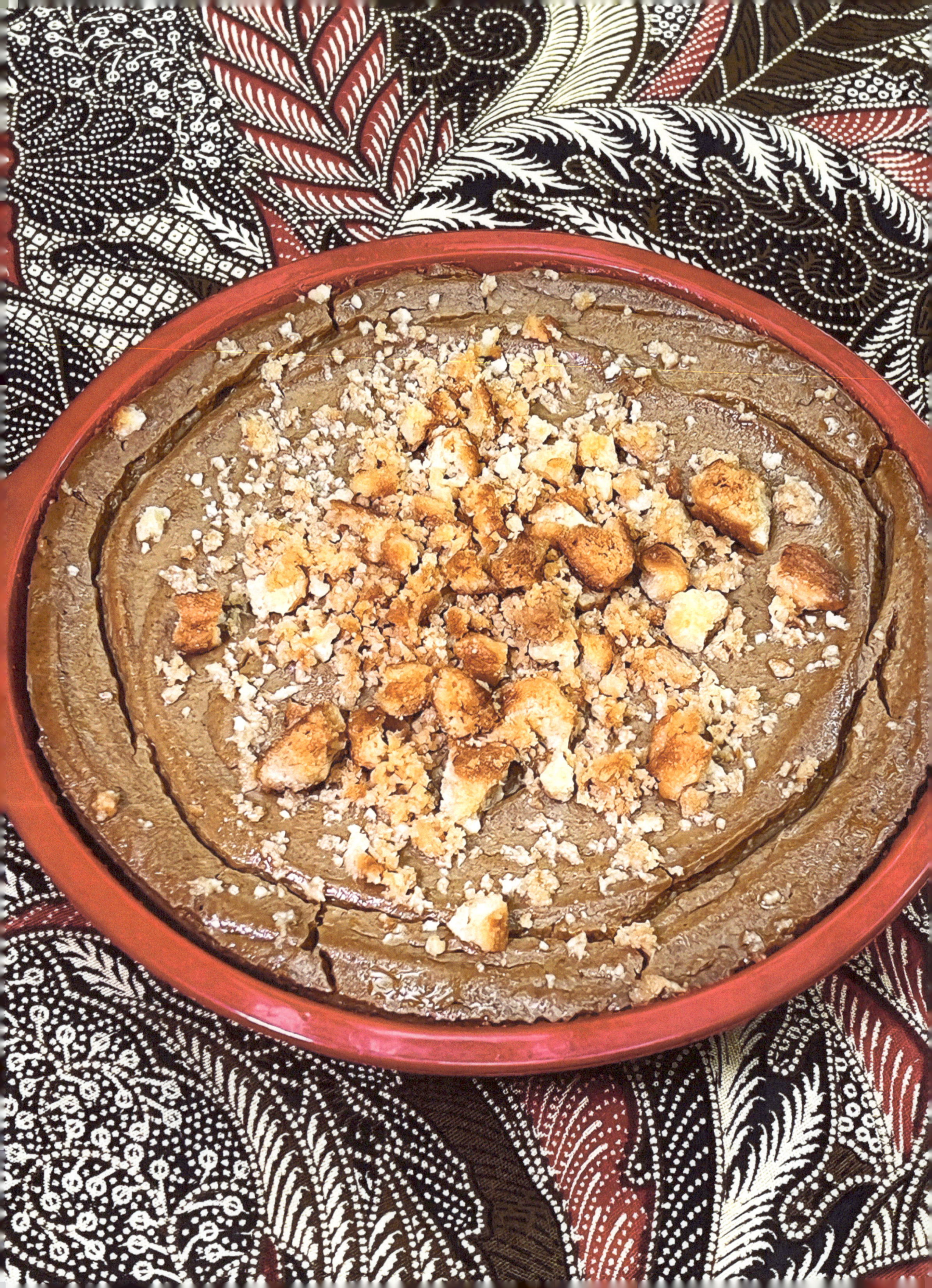

TOFU PUMPKIN PIE

I once did a blind taste test between this vegan recipe and the classic Joy of Cooking pumpkin pie recipe, which includes heaps of rich cream and eggs. The tasters were two guys who were anything but vegan. They both liked the vegan version best. Nuff said.

INGREDIENTS

◇◇◇◇◇◇◇◇◇◇◇◇◇

Crust
- 2 cups graham crackers or ginger snaps, crushed into crumbs
- 1/3 cup solid fat

Filling
- 2 cups cooked pumpkin (one large 15 oz can)
- 1 container firm silken tofu
- 1 cup sugar
- 1 Tbsp pumpkin spice powder
  – Or 1 tsp each allspice, cinnamon, and ginger powder + a pinch of clove and nutmeg
- 1/4 tsp salt

INSTRUCTIONS

◇◇◇◇◇◇◇◇◇◇◇◇◇

1. Mix the fat with cookie crumbs until combined.
2. Press the crumb mixture into a pie pan and I mean press!
3. Blend the filling ingredients in a food processor or with a hand blender until completely smooth.
4. Pour the filling into the crust and bake at 350°F until set, about 45 minutes.
5. Allow to cool before serving with whipped cream or ice cream.

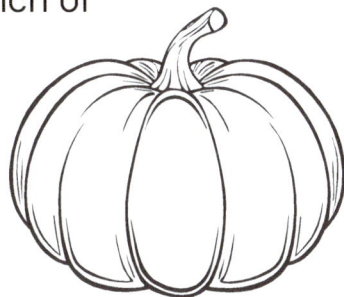

Notes:

Another crust solution is to make **Any Shape Lemon Cookies** and substitute water or milk for the lemon juice. Roll out and place in a greased pie pan (or press into place). Bake for 10 minutes. Fill and bake again until filling is set. You can also buy a premade pie crust from the store, which is cheating, but your secret is safe with me.

vegan

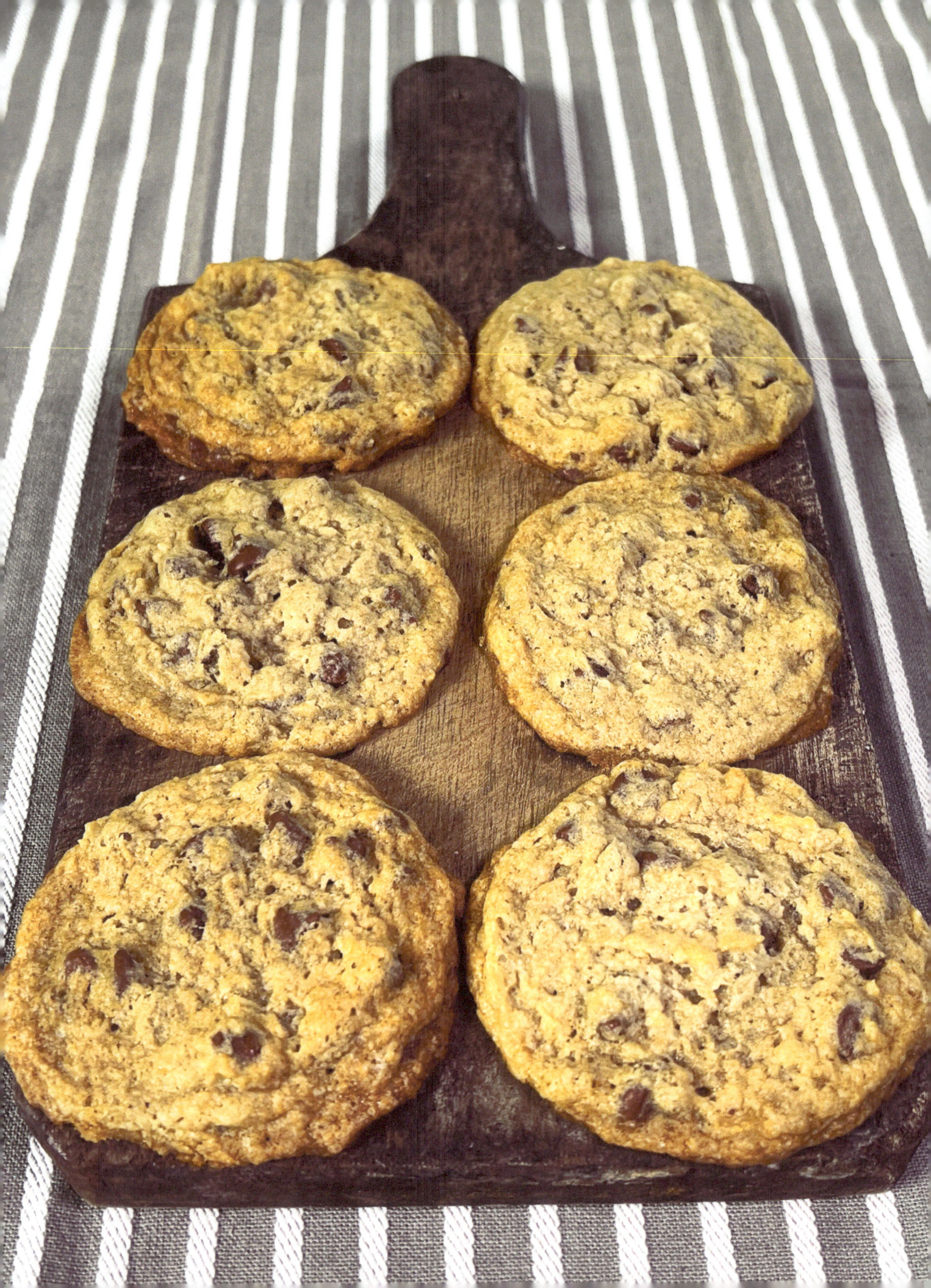

ALMOST CLASSIC CHOCOLATE CHIP COOKIES

When served hot from the oven, while the chocolate chips are still melty, these cookies are a classic experience. If you use dairy-free chocolate chips they are #vegan, otherwise they are #mostlyvegan.

INGREDIENTS

◇◇◇◇◇◇◇◇◇◇◇◇

Dry
- 2 cups flour
- 1 tsp baking soda
- 1 cup chocolate chips

Wet
- 3/4 cup solid fat
- 1 cup light brown or raw sugar
- 1 Tbsp vanilla
- 1 ripe banana
- 1/2 tsp salt

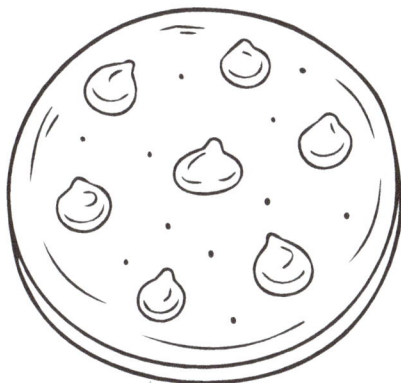

INSTRUCTIONS

◇◇◇◇◇◇◇◇◇◇◇◇

1. Mix the dry ingredients completely.
2. Blend the wet ingredients until creamy.
3. Combine the wet and dry ingredients, gently stirring so the chocolate chips are evenly distributed and each cookie gets a fair shake.
4. Scoop the cookie dough onto your well-greased baking sheet. Space them apart enough to let them spread while baking.
5. Bake at 350°F until the delicious smell of baking cookies fills the air and the cookies are brown on the edges, about 10 minutes.

vegan

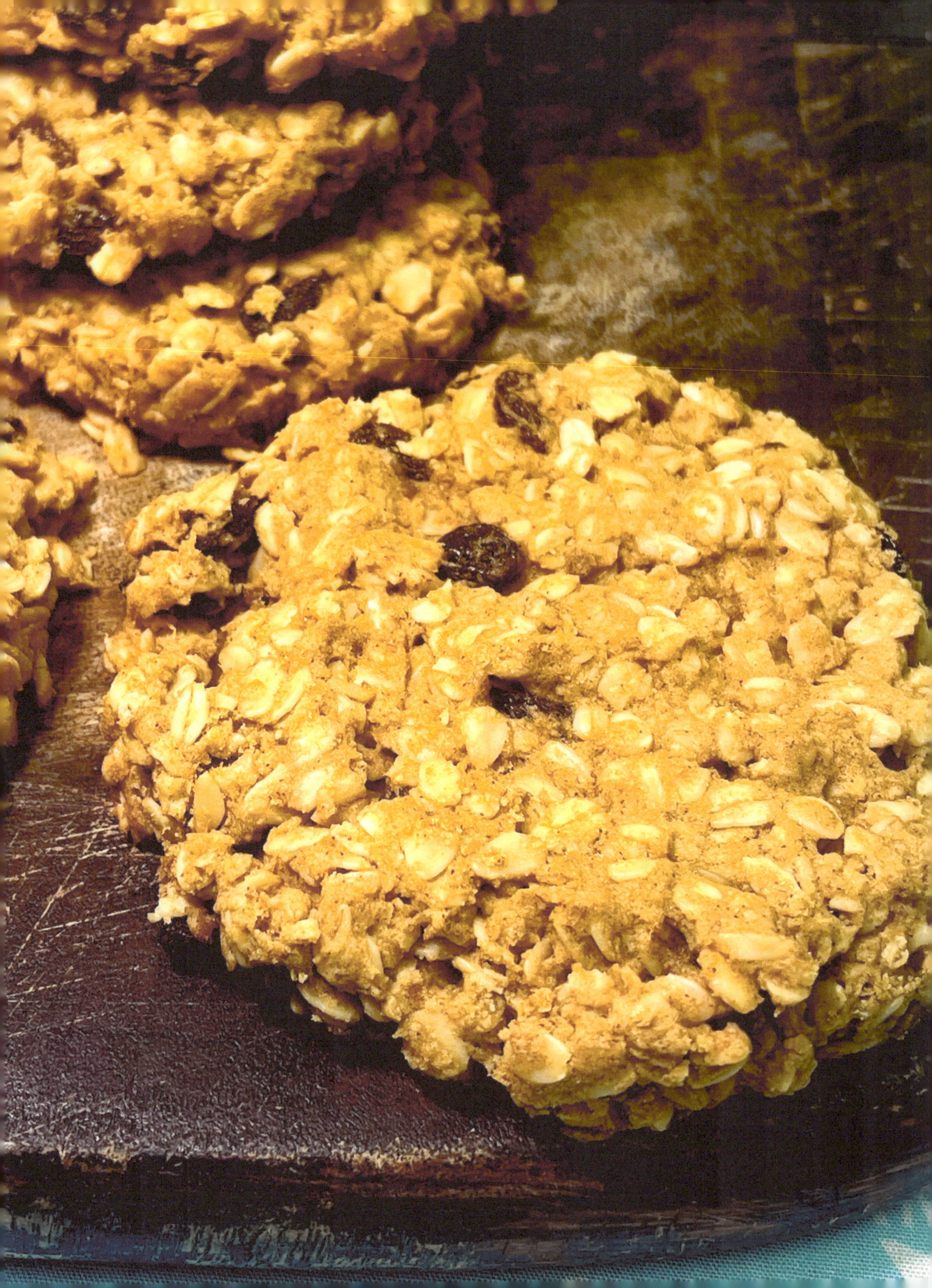

OLD-FASHIONED OATMEAL RAISIN COOKIES

I simplified the classic recipe and beefed up the whole oats component for you. The result is a hearty cookie that is just a little on the dry side, like a good sense of humor.

INGREDIENTS
◇◇◇◇◇◇◇◇◇◇◇◇

Dry
- 1½ cups flour
- 1 tsp baking soda
- 1/2 tsp baking powder
- 1/2 tsp salt
- 1 Tbsp cinnamon
- 3 cups old-fashioned oats (NOT quick oats)
- 1 cup raisins

Wet
- 1 cup light brown or raw sugar
- 3/4 cup solid fat
- 1 tsp vanilla
- 1 ripe banana

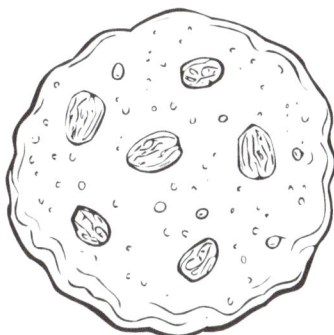

INSTRUCTIONS
◇◇◇◇◇◇◇◇◇◇◇◇

1. Mix the dry ingredients completely.
2. Blend the wet ingredients until creamy.
3. Combine the wet and dry ingredients. At first, it may be hard to believe that there will be enough wet stuff to absorb all the dry. If you're willing to get your hands dirty, go ahead and dig in there. You'll see, it all comes together.
4. Scoop the cookie dough onto your well-greased baking sheet and smash down into shape, as these cookies don't spread much.
5. Bake at 350°F until the warm smell of cookies permeates the air and the edges of the cookies are brown, about 8 minutes.

Notes:

You can replace the chocolate chips for raisins to make a chewy, gooey, chocolatey treat.

Vegan

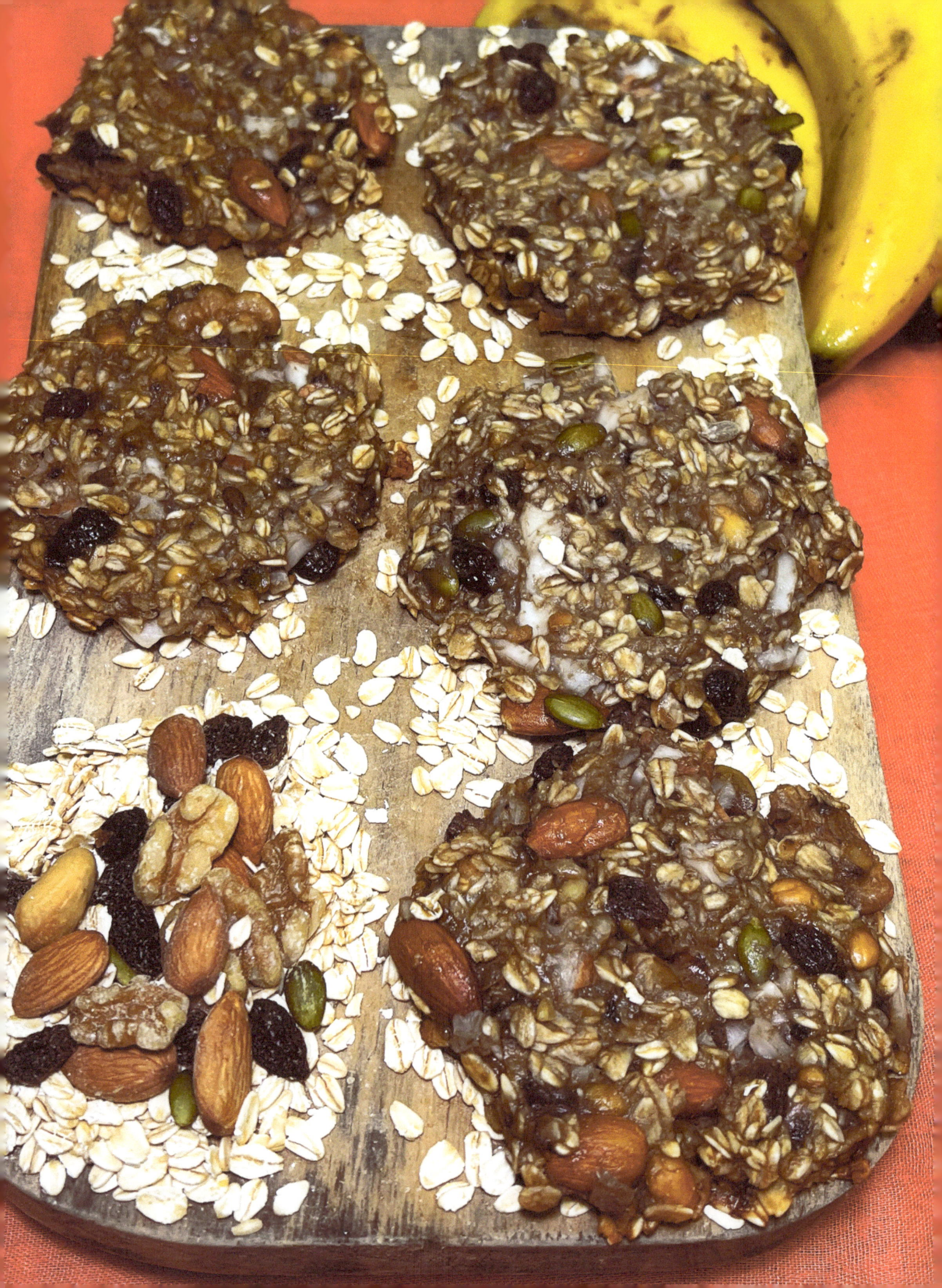

FREE COOKIES!

Sugar-free, dairy-free, wheat-free, and fat-free. These cookies are simple and nutritious enough to eat for breakfast... guilt-free!

INGREDIENTS

◇◇◇◇◇◇◇◇◇◇◇◇

Necessary
- 5-7 ripe bananas (~ 1 $\frac{1}{3}$ lbs)
- 3 cups old-fashioned oats (NOT quick oats)

Optional
- Raisins or dried cranberries
- Nuts of any kind. Mix 'em up!
- Chocolate chips
- Peanut butter
- Spices like cinnamon and ginger

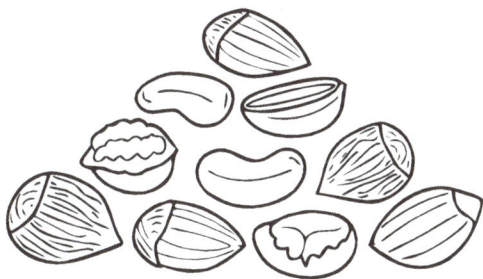

INSTRUCTIONS

◇◇◇◇◇◇◇◇◇◇◇◇

1. Peel the bananas and toss them into a big bowl.
2. Mush the bananas using an electric mixer or squish them with your hands.
3. Dump the oats along with any optional ingredients into the bowl with the bananas and smush everything together.
4. Scoop lumps of dough onto well-greased baking sheets and form into whatever shapes you please. You can use an ice cream scoop to make tidy hills, flatten them into discs, or leave them as loosey-goosey as you like.
5. Bake at 350°F until the natural sugar in the bananas begins to caramelize, about 25 minutes.

Notes:
The only two essential ingredients are bananas and oats – have fun improvising from there!

vegan

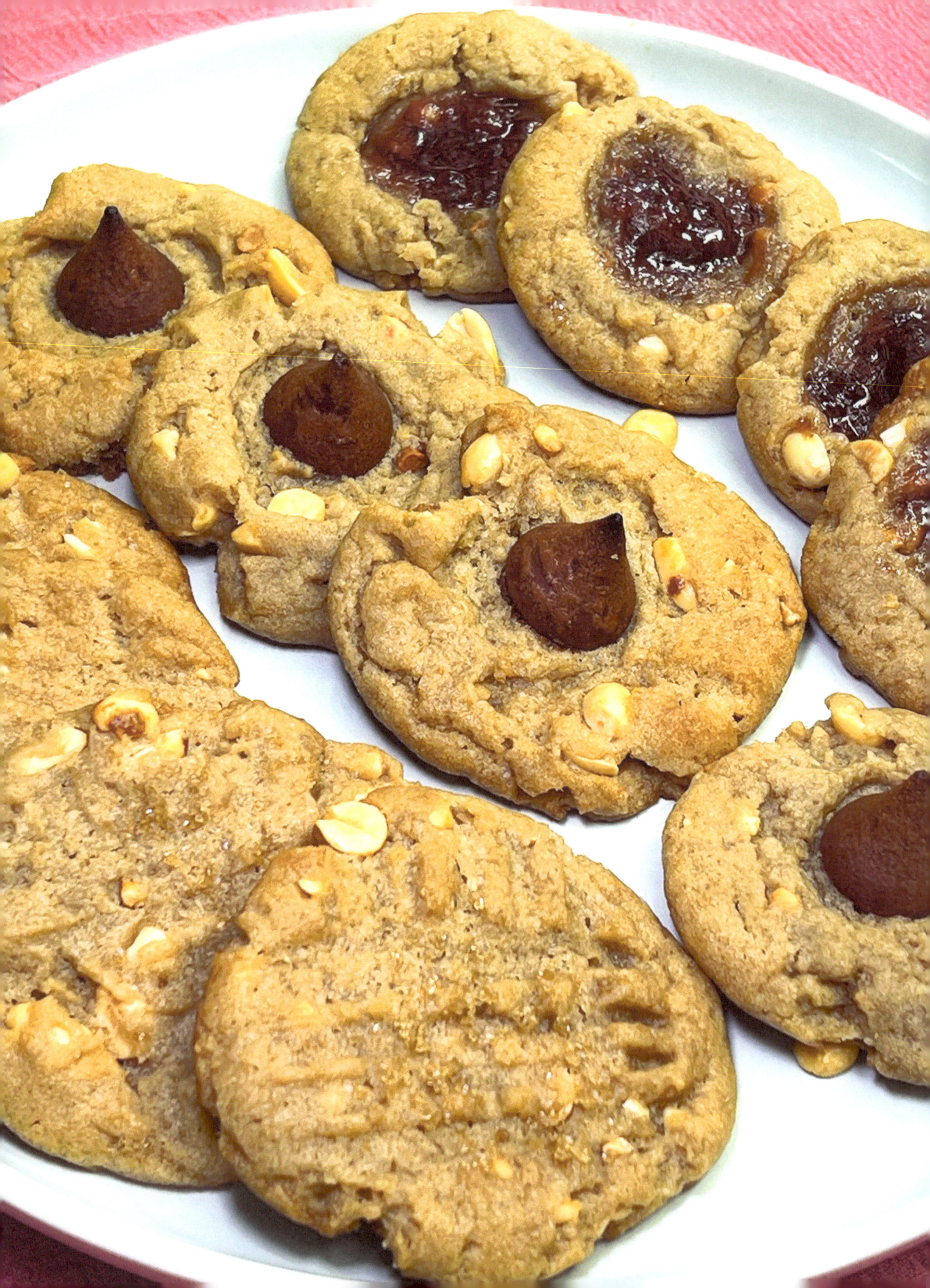

EXTRA CRUNCHY
PEANUT BUTTER COOKIES

The addition of peanuts makes these cookies not just crunchy – they're extra crunchy!

INGREDIENTS

◇◇◇◇◇◇◇◇◇◇◇◇

Dry
- 2 cups flour
- 1 tsp baking soda
- 1/2 tsp salt
- 1 cup peanuts

Wet
- 1 cup light brown sugar
- 1/2 cup solid fat
- 3/4 cup peanut butter
- 1 Tbsp vanilla
- 1 banana

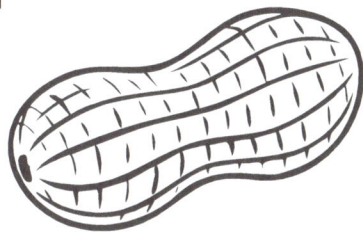

INSTRUCTIONS

◇◇◇◇◇◇◇◇◇◇◇◇

1. Mix the dry ingredients completely.
2. Blend the wet ingredients until creamy.
3. Combine the wet and dry ingredients.
4. Form the dough into balls with your hands and place onto lightly oiled baking sheets. Press down on the dough with the tines of a fork to create the classic crosshatch pattern, then sprinkle with cinnamon–sugar.
5. Bake at 350°F until the cookies are barely browned on the edges, about 10 minutes. Beware that these cookies burn easily!

Notes:
- If you use salted peanuts, omit the salt in the recipe, unless you are going for a sweet & salty kind of thing.
- For a Reese's Peanut Butter Cup cookie, press a Hershey's Kiss into the center of each dough ball.
- For a PB&J cookie, press your thumb into the center of each dough ball to create an indentation, then fill it with jam or jelly.
- For a totally decadent treat, add some chocolate chips to make Peanut Butter Chocolate Chip Cookies.

Vegan

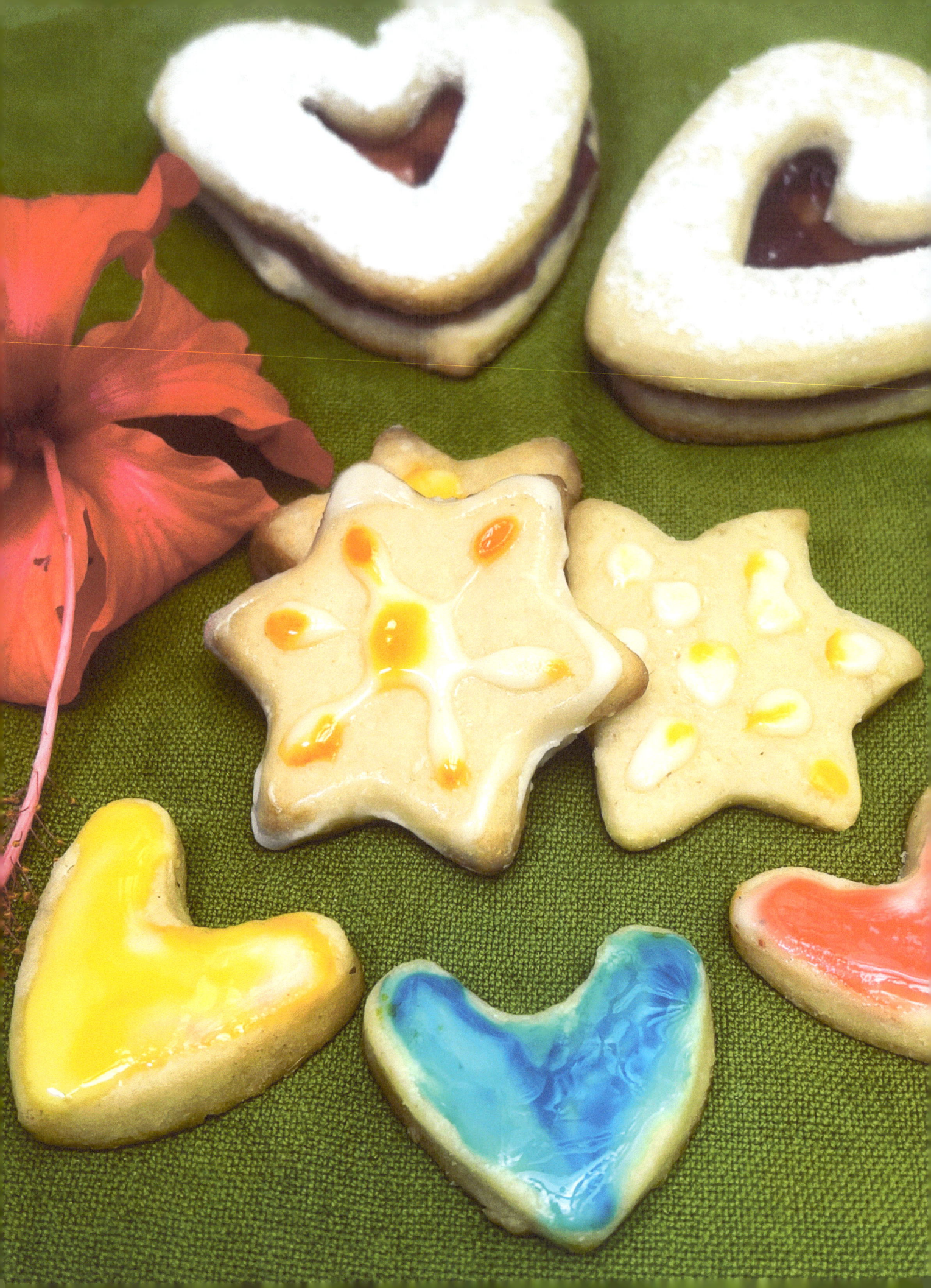

ANY SHAPE LEMON COOKIES

Deliciously simple sugar cookies with a surprising lemon twist. Form them into any shape that fulfills your creative wishes.

INGREDIENTS

◇◇◇◇◇◇◇◇◇◇◇◇◇

Dry
- 2 ½ cups flour

Wet
- 1 cup solid fat
- 2/3 cup white sugar
- 1 tsp vanilla
- 1/2 tsp salt
- 1/2 cup lemon juice
- 1 Tbsp lemon zest (if available)
- 1 Tbsp flax meal

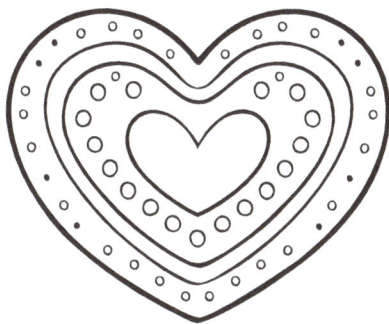

INSTRUCTIONS

◇◇◇◇◇◇◇◇◇◇◇◇◇

1. Blend the wet ingredients until creamy.
2. Add the flour and mix well.
3. The dough will be firm yet soft. Form it into a ball and chill in the fridge for at least two hours. If you're in a hurry, you can chill it in the freezer for an hour.
4. Roll out the dough on a floured or nonstick surface, such as silicone baking sheets or waxed paper, to desired cookie thickness, 1/4 – 1/2 inch.
5. Cut into any shape you like using cookie cutters or a knife.
6. Place on baking sheets and bake at 350°F until the edges just hint at brown, about 8 minutes.

Decoration Notes:
- Frost cooled cookies with **Sweet Tart Lemon Icing**
  OR – sprinkle with colored sugar or crushed candy before baking.
- For tarts, make matching cookie pairs, one with a center cutout. After baking, cover the full cookie with jam, sift powdered sugar onto the cutout cookie, and then sandwich the two together. Yum!

Vegan

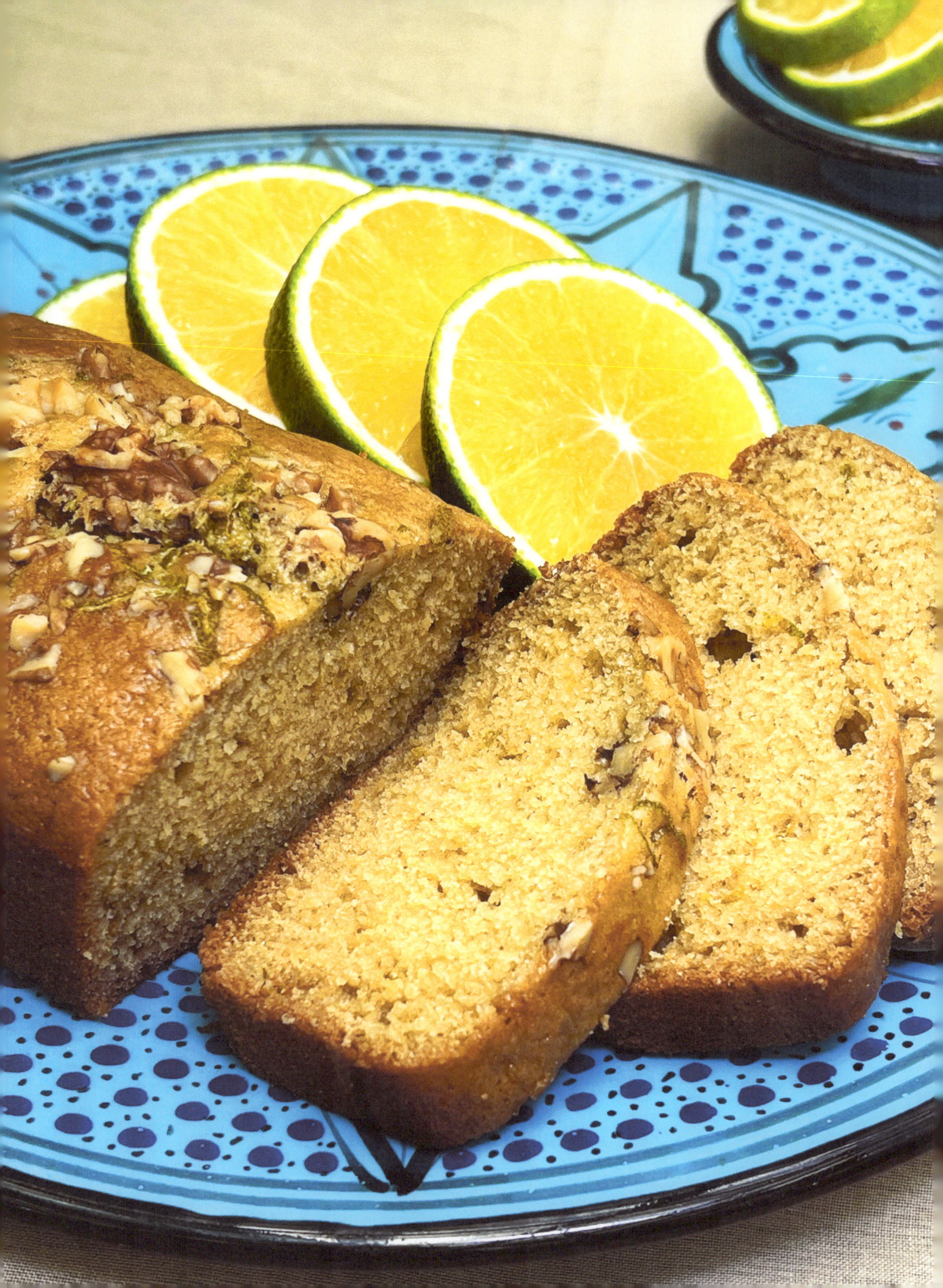

GRANDMA'S ORANGE BREAD

My grandmother has an orange tree in the backyard of her house in Orange County, California. When she has more oranges than she knows what to do with, she juices them and bakes this lightly sweet orange bread. As a kid, I would toast thick slices and slather them with butter and jam to make a tasty after-school snack.

INGREDIENTS

◇◇◇◇◇◇◇◇◇◇◇◇

Dry
- 2 cups flour
- 1 tsp baking soda
- 1 tsp baking powder
- 1/4 tsp salt
- 1/4 tsp cardamom or ginger powder

Wet
- Grated rind of one orange
- 1 cup orange juice
  – fresh squeezed is best
- 1 cup sugar
- 2 Tbsp vegetable oil
- 1 egg
- 1 tsp vanilla

Optional additions
- 1/2 cup raisins
- 1/2 cup walnuts

INSTRUCTIONS

◇◇◇◇◇◇◇◇◇◇◇◇

1. Mix the dry ingredients until evenly combined.
2. Stir the wet ingredients together.
3. Combine the wet and dry ingredients.
4. Scoop the batter into a greased and floured bread pan.
5. Bake at 350°F until a toothpick inserted in the center comes out clean, about 45 minutes.

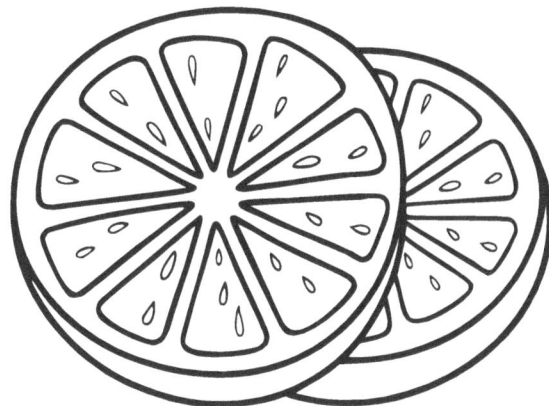

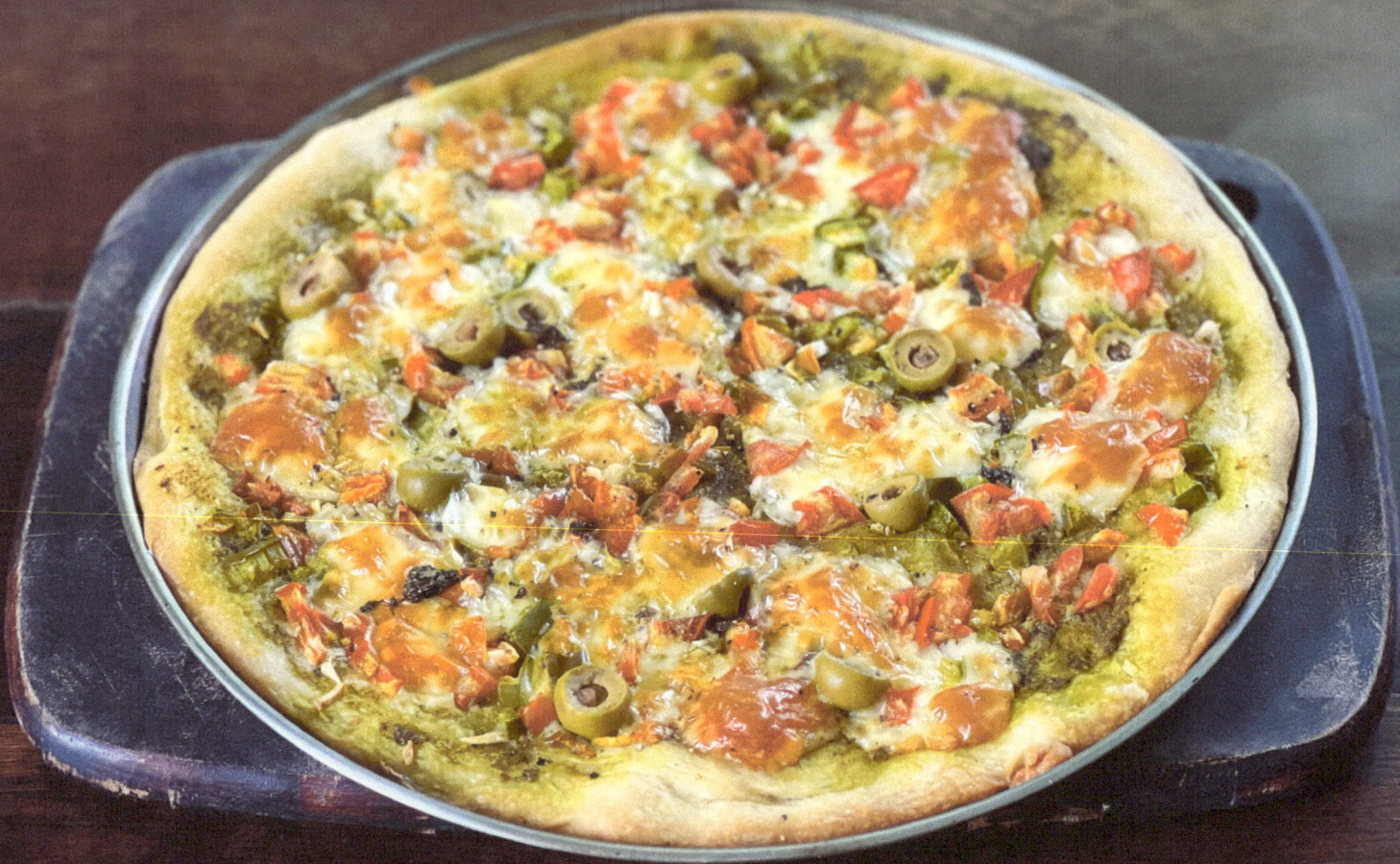

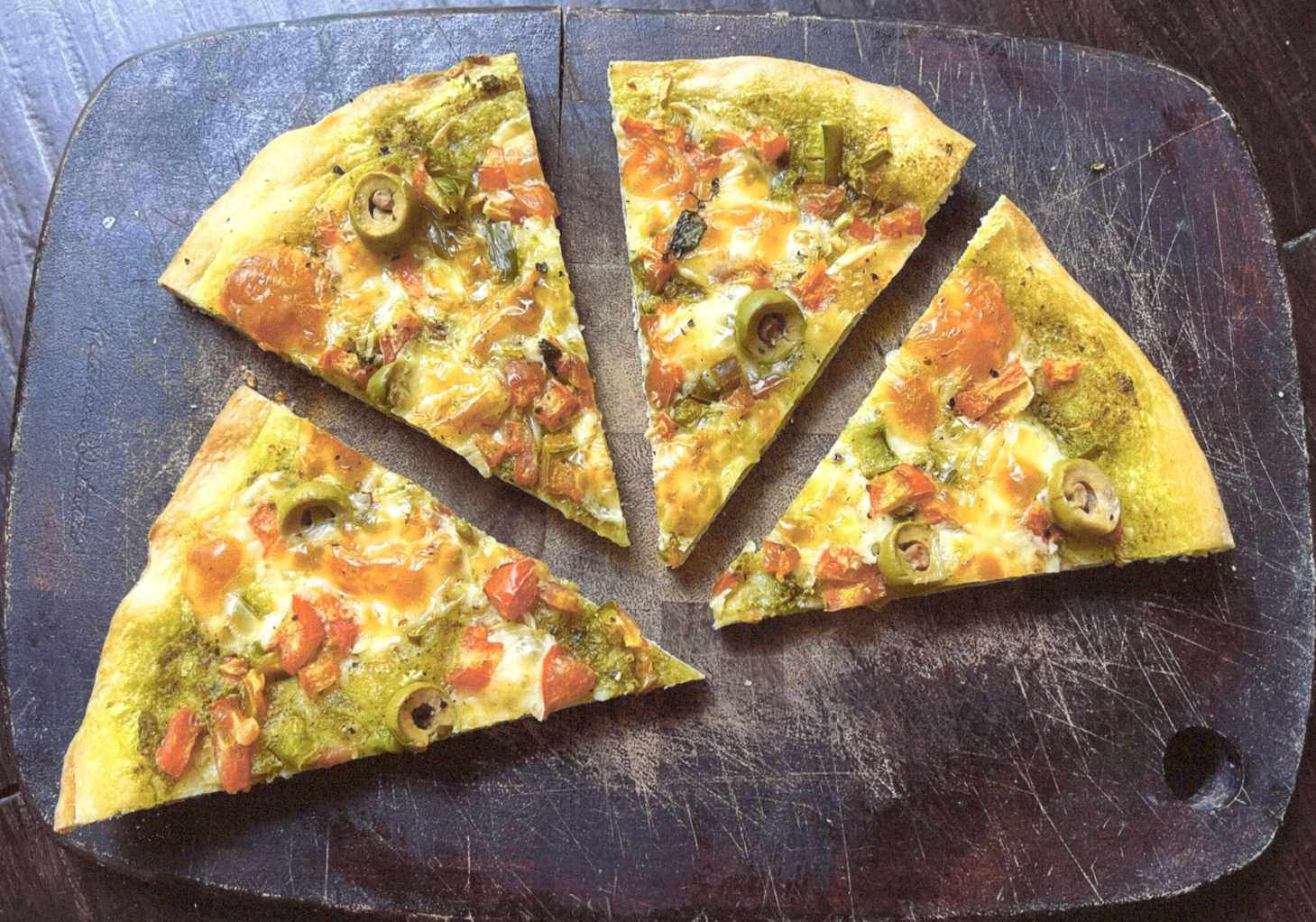

QUICK & EASY PIZZA DOUGH

INGREDIENTS

◇◇◇◇◇◇◇◇◇◇◇◇◇

- 3 cups flour
- 1 tsp salt
- 1 tsp sugar
- 1 Tbsp yeast
- 1 cup water
- 3 Tbsp olive oil

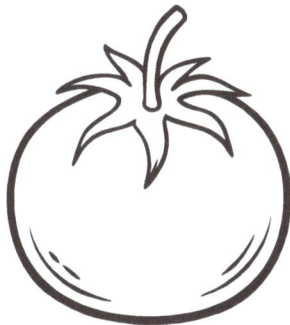

INSTRUCTIONS

◇◇◇◇◇◇◇◇◇◇◇◇◇

1. Put everything into a big bowl and mix it up with your hands.
2. Knead the dough for a few minutes, adding more flour as needed to keep it from sticking to your hands.
3. Form the dough into a ball and drizzle with olive oil to keep it from sticking to the bowl. Cover and let it rise for 10-20 minutes while you prep the toppings.
4. Pat, roll, or toss the dough into shape and place on oiled pizza pan.
5. Add your toppings.
6. Bake at 400°F until the crust is well-browned on the edges, about 25 minutes.

Notes:
- Mix and knead the dough right in the bowl for easy cleanup.
- The rising time is flexible. If you're in a rush, you can shape, top, and bake it right away. If you need more time to prepare a fantastic sauce, let it rise longer—just be sure to punch it down from time to time.
- One trick to avoid soggy crusts is to coat the dough with olive oil before adding other toppings. Also, go easy on the wet ingredients like fresh tomatoes, or cook them before putting on the pizza.
- Make a few batches of this recipe at a time, form them into pizza-sized balls, put them in plastic bags, and freeze. Just toss them in the fridge to thaw in the morning, and you'll be set for your pizza party tonight!

Vegan

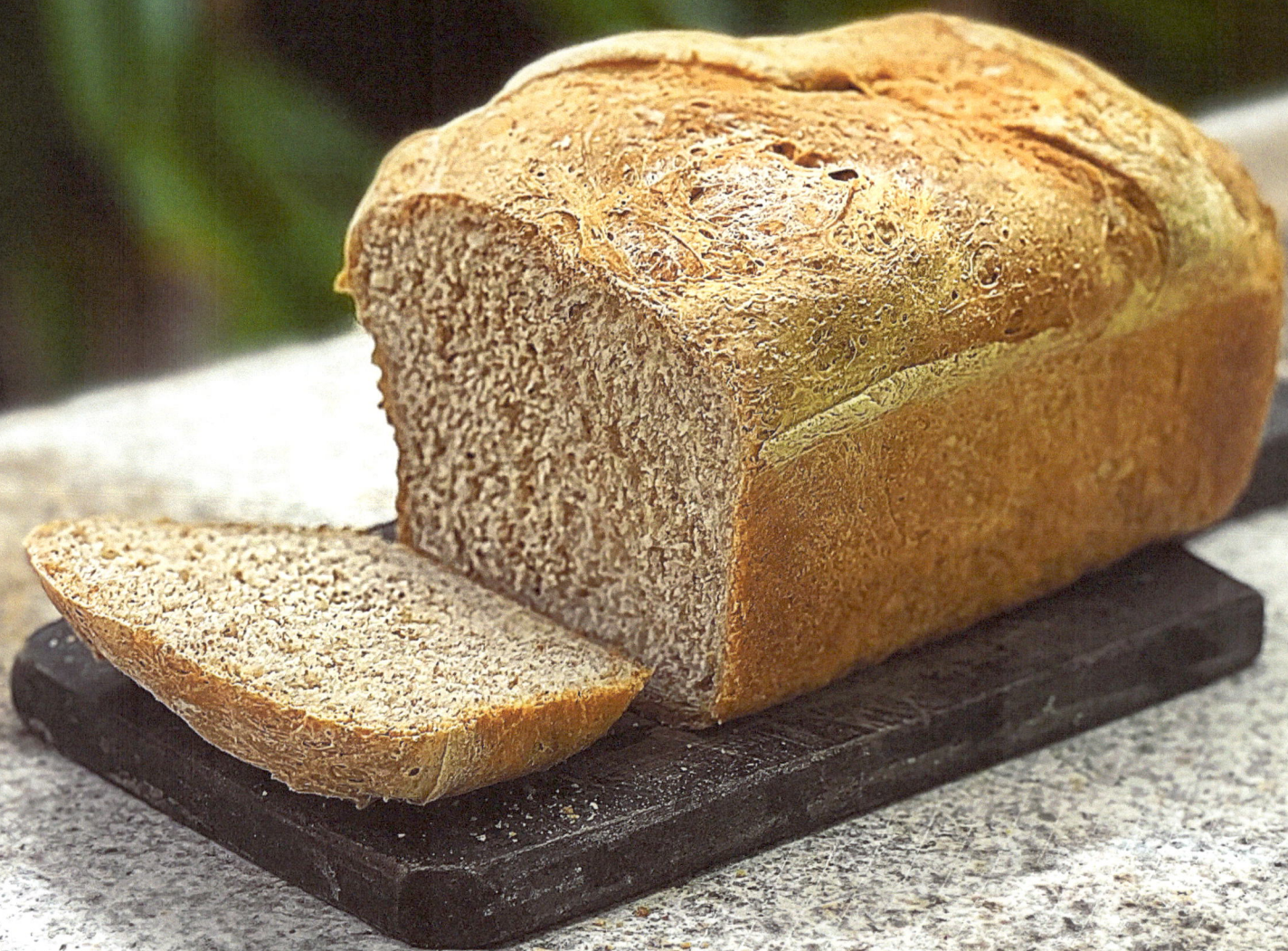

WHOLESOME WHOLE WHEAT BREAD

Is there anything cozier than homemade bread hot from the oven? How about a healthy whole wheat version? This recipe makes 2 good-sized loaves, 4 small loaves, or a whole bunch of buns.

INGREDIENTS

◇◇◇◇◇◇◇◇◇◇◇◇

- 6 cups whole wheat flour + more flour for kneading
- 1 tsp salt
- 2 Tbsp sugar
- 2 Tbsp yeast
- 4 Tbsp oil
- 4 cups water

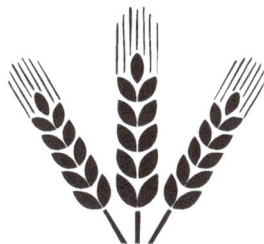

INSTRUCTIONS

◇◇◇◇◇◇◇◇◇◇◇◇

1. Place 6 cups of flour and the other ingredients in a big bowl and stir together with a big spoon. The dough will be gooey. Cover and let rest for 60 minutes.
2. Come back to the dough when it's about twice the size, about 30 minutes. Add a couple more cups of flour and use your hands to pull the dough in from the edges of the bowl. Keep adding more flour, one handful at a time, just enough to keep your hands from sticking, turning the bowl as you go. Knead for 5 minutes, about the length of a song.
3. Drizzle on some oil. Turn the dough to coat it on both sides to prevent sticking to the bowl. Cover and let rise for another 45 minutes or so.
4. Punch down the dough with a satisfying "Hah!".
5. Let it rest for about 10 minutes before shaping the dough into the form you like (loaf, ball, rolls, bread sticks, braids, etc.).
6. Let it rise again for about 30 minutes.
7. Bake at 350°F until the delectable smell of fresh baked bread pervades your senses and the crust is golden brown, about 45 minutes.

vegan

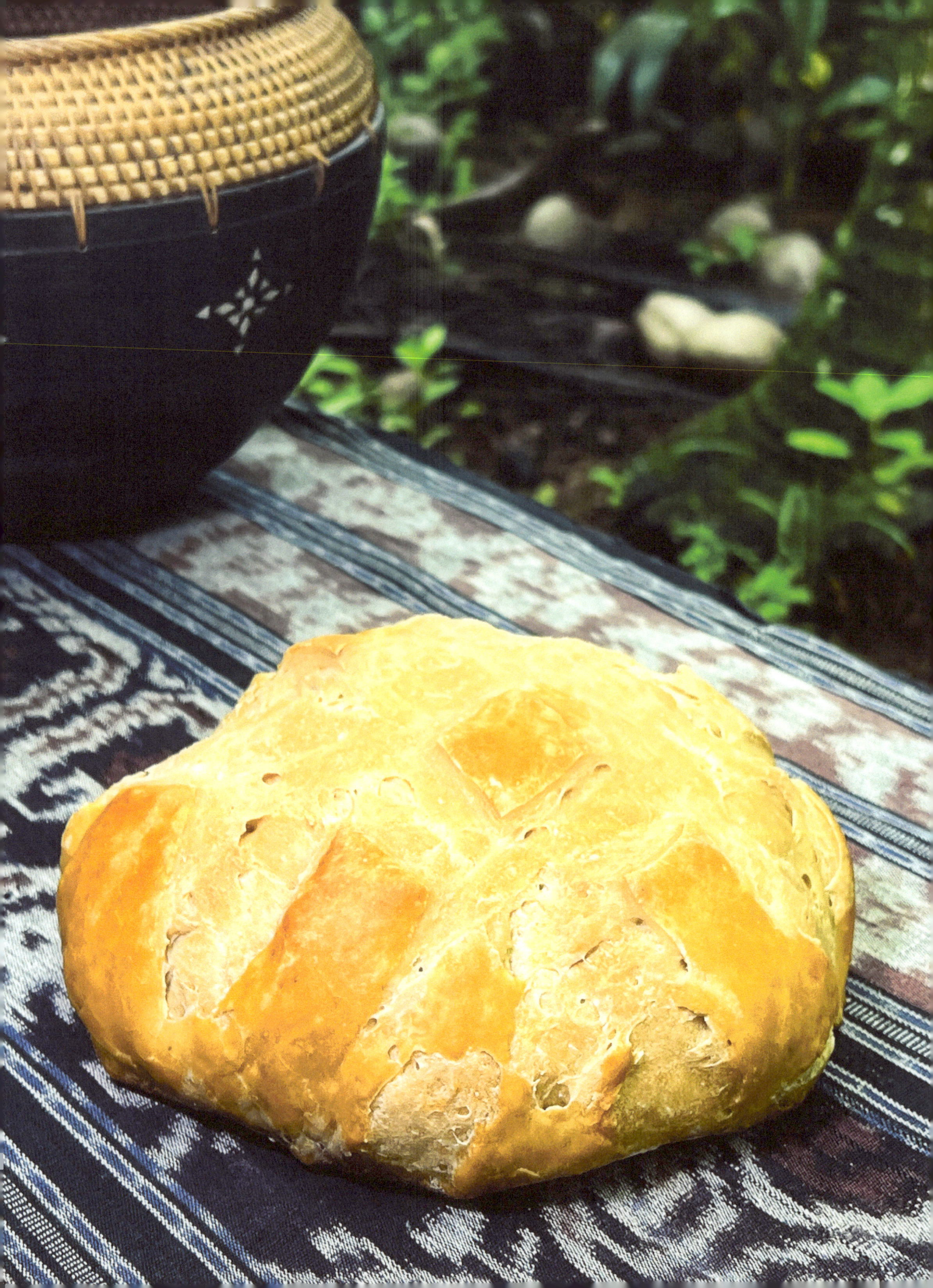

SOURDOUGH BREAD DEMYSTIFIED

Are you afraid of making sourdough bread? You are not alone, so was I. The recipes I read sounded like I needed an advanced degree in chemistry. Now I know that sourdough bread, like life, can actually be pretty easy.

STARTER

INGREDIENTS

- 1 cup flour
- 1/2 cup water
- 1 tsp yeast

INSTRUCTIONS

1. Mix the starter ingredients in a jar that is big enough for the starter to rise to about 2x the volume without overflowing. A quart-size bell jar works great. Cover it loosely with a cloth to keep the bugs out and leave it on the counter in a convenient place.
2. Every day, dump out half of the starter and stir in 1 cup of flour and ½ cup of water. Think of it like feeding a pet. It's ready to use when it smells sour, typically within a few days to a week.

DOUGH

INGREDIENTS

- 2 + 3 cups flour
- 1 cup starter
- 1 cup water
- 1 tsp yeast
- 1 tsp salt
- 1 Tbsp oil

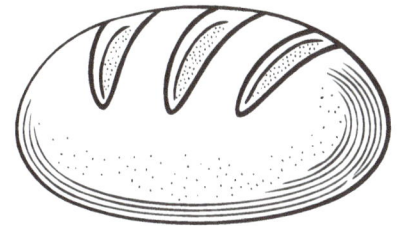

INSTRUCTIONS

1. Mix the ingredients in a large container, ideally one with straight sides, so you can easily see how much the dough has risen.
2. Mark the side of the container at the dough's starting height. Let it rise until doubled, but no more! This can take anywhere from 1-4 hours.
3. Punch down, add 2-3 more cups of flour, and knead until smooth.
4. Let rise until doubled again.
5. Punch down, shape, and place on a baking tray or in a loaf pan.
6. Slice the top in a fun way, then bake at 350°F until the crust is golden brown, about 45 minutes.

Vegan

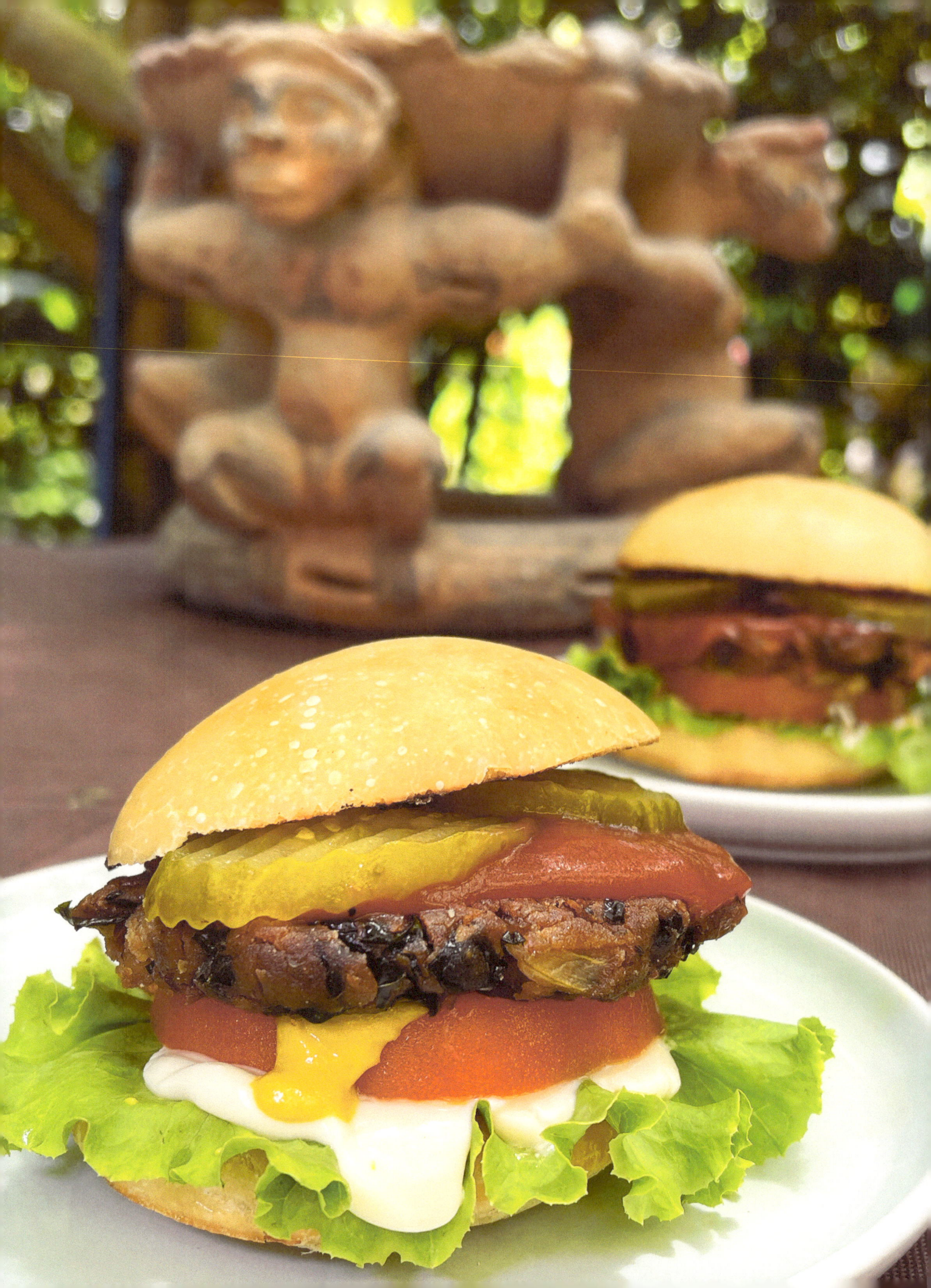

MESOAMERICAN VEGGIE BURGERS

Named after the three staple foods of ancient Central (Meso) America —beans, corn (maize), and squash— these foods were traditionally grown together in a productive intercropping system that supported a thriving population since pre-Columbian times. Today, we can enjoy how well these three nutritious foods taste together in a vegan burger. You can use any kind of hard squash, such as pumpkin, acorn, or butternut squash. Avoid watery squashes like zucchini, as they can make the dough too wet.

INGREDIENTS

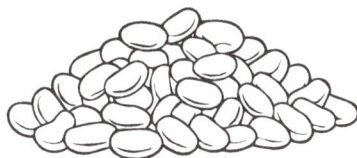

- 2 cups cooked beans (a 19 oz can)
- 2/3 cup corn/maize tortilla flour (masa)
- 2/3 cup chopped winter squash
- 2/3 cup chopped onion
- 2/3 cup chopped greens
- 1/4 cup oil
- 1 tsp salt
- 1 tsp cumin powder
- 1 tsp dry oregano
- 1 tsp cayenne powder
- 1 Tbsp soy sauce
- Lizano or BBQ sauce for glaze

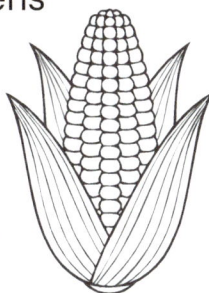

INSTRUCTIONS

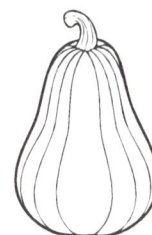

1. Soak, cook, and drain beans, or use drained canned beans.
2. Chop veggies into pieces roughly the same size as the beans.
3. Mix all the ingredients together and knead with your hands into a stiff dough.
4. Coat your baking sheet with a generous amount of oil.
5. Scoop out handfuls of dough and form into 4-6 patties.
6. Brush the patties with sauce or oil.
7. Bake at 350°F until they begin to get a bit brown, about 35 minutes.
8. Enjoy straight from the oven or fry in oil until crispy.

Vegan

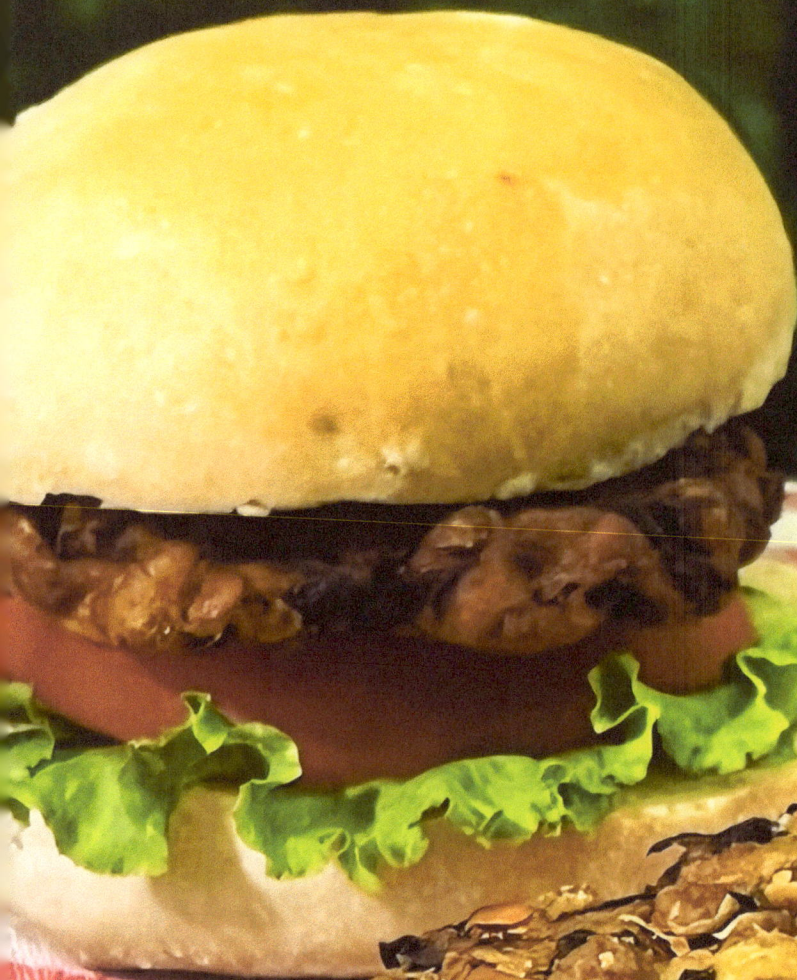

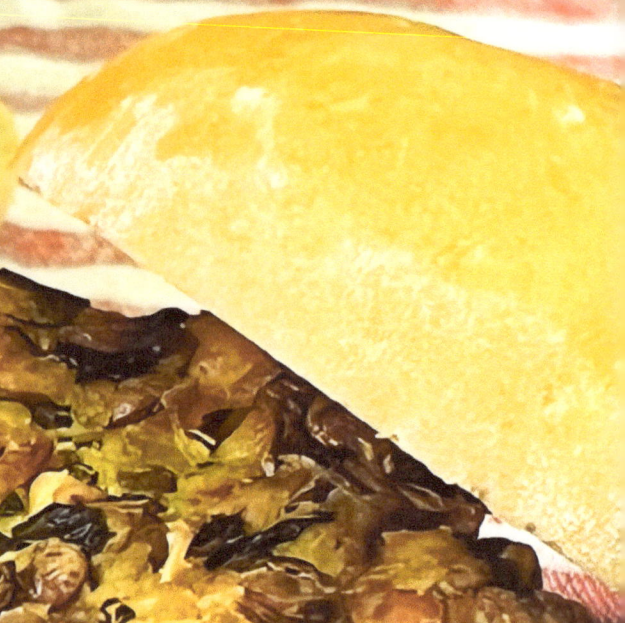

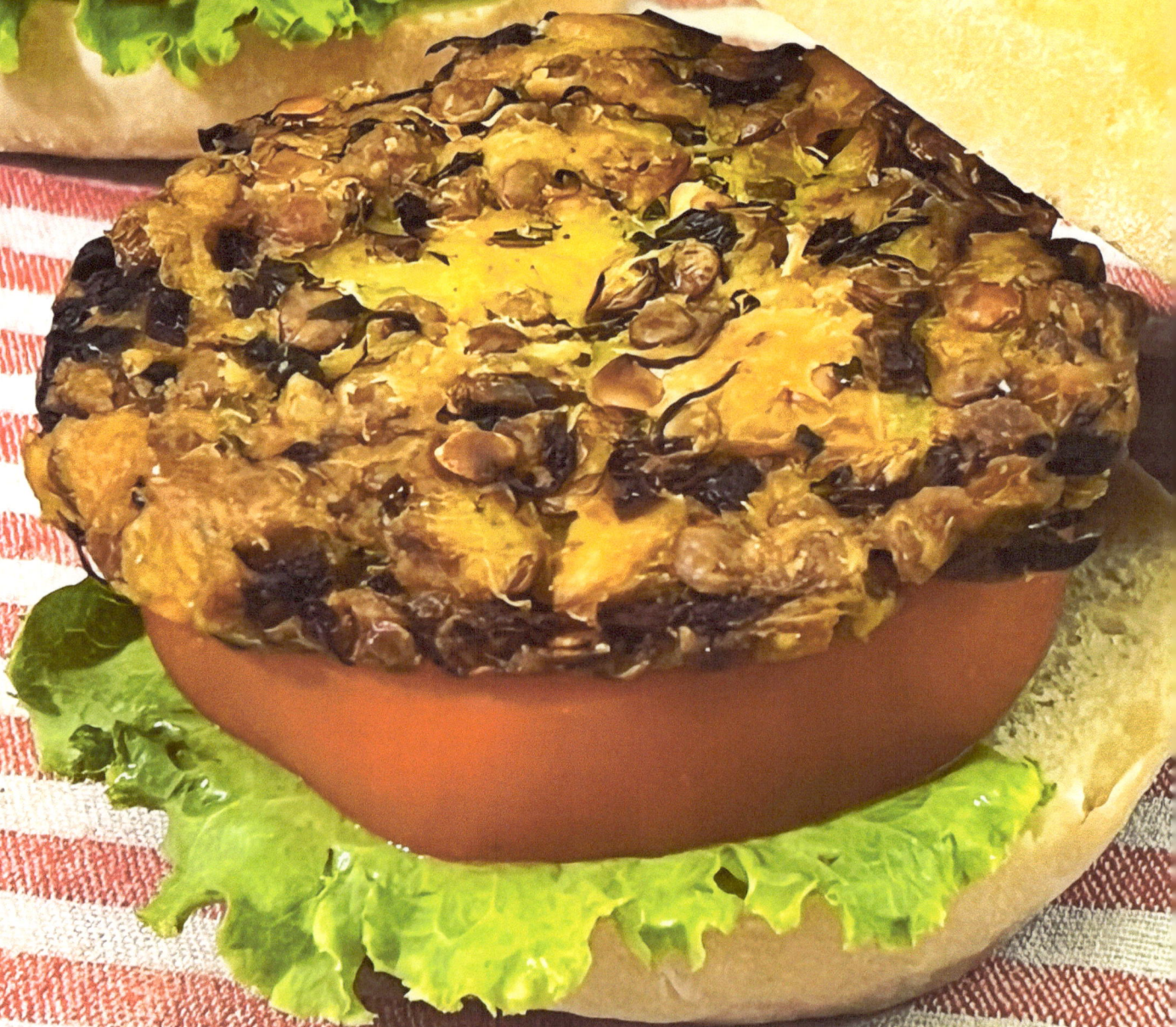

SPROUTED LENTIL CURRY VEGGIE BURGERS

It took me many tries to find a way to make sprouted lentils stick together, and cooked yucca does the trick! Also known as manioc or cassava, yucca is a staple food in many parts of the world. In addition to its binding power, it adds a subtle sweetness and fries to a perfect crisp.

INGREDIENTS

◇◇◇◇◇◇◇◇◇◇◇◇◇

- 1 cup sprouted lentils
- 1/3 cup finely chopped onions
- 1/3 cup grated carrot
- 1/4 cup finely chopped greens
- 1 clove minced garlic
- 1/2 tsp salt
- 1/4 tsp black pepper
- 1 tsp curry powder
- 3 Tbsp oil
- 1 cup cooked, cooled, and smushed yucca root

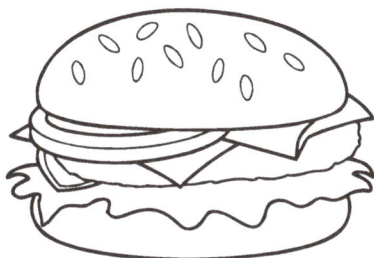

INSTRUCTIONS

◇◇◇◇◇◇◇◇◇◇◇◇◇

1. Sprout the lentils: soak whole lentils overnight in water, drain, and place in a sunny spot for 2–4 days until they sprout. Rinse daily to keep them moist.
2. Cook the yucca: peel, chop, and boil until soft, about 20 minutes.
3. Mix everything but the yucca in a large bowl.
4. Add yucca and mash everything together with your hands.
5. Form into 4–6 patties and bake at 350°F on a greased baking sheet until they start to brown, approximately 25 minutes.
6. Enjoy straight from the oven or fry in oil until crispy.

Notes:
Double or triple the recipe to have plenty for later! Layer the baked burgers with squares of waxed paper, place them in a sealed plastic bag, and freeze.

Vegan

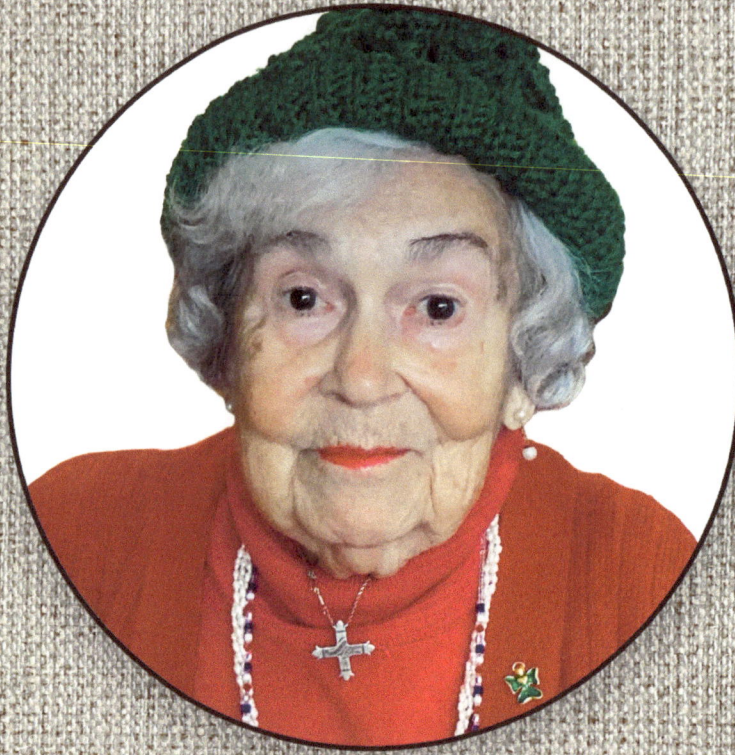

This cookbook
is dedicated to
Grandma Carol.